With best wishes

Plastic Surgery in Wars, Disasters and Civilian Life

Dedication

To Vivian – my wife, friend and supporter for fifty years.
And to my daughters Clare and Natasha – who saw me
only occasionally during their early years.

The income from this book will be donated to
'Restore – Burn and Wound Research',
a medical research charity that I set up thirty years ago.

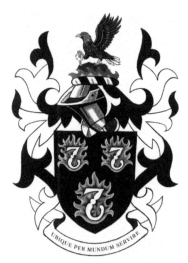

The Arms and Crest of
Professor Anthony Roberts
OBE OStJ

Plastic Surgery in Wars, Disasters and Civilian Life

The Memoirs of
Professor Anthony H.N. Roberts
OBE, OStJ, MA, BSc, BM, BCh, FRCS,
FRCSG, FRSB, FRGS

Anthony Roberts

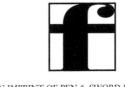

AN IMPRINT OF PEN & SWORD BOOKS LTD
YORKSHIRE – PHILADELPHIA

First published in Great Britain in 2023 by
FRONTLINE BOOKS
an imprint of Pen & Sword Books Ltd
Yorkshire – Philadelphia

Copyright © Anthony Roberts, 2023

ISBN 9-781-39906-848-2

The right of Anthony Roberts to be identified as the author of this work has been asserted by him in accordance with the Copyright, Designs and Patents Act 1988.

A CIP catalogue record for this book is available from the British Library.

All rights reserved. No part of this book may be reproduced or transmitted in any form or by any means, electronic or mechanical including photocopying, recording or by any information storage and retrieval system, without permission from the Publisher in writing.

Typeset by Concept, Huddersfield, West Yorkshire, HD4 5JL.
Printed on paper from a sustainable source by CPI Group (UK) Ltd,
Croydon CR0 4YY.

Pen & Sword Books Ltd incorporates the imprints of Aviation, Atlas, Family History, Fiction, Maritime, Military, Discovery, Politics, History, Archaeology, Select, Wharncliffe Local History, Wharncliffe True Crime, Military Classics, Wharncliffe Transport, Leo Cooper, The Praetorian Press, Remember When, White Owl, Seaforth Publishing and Frontline Books.

For a complete list of Pen & Sword titles please contact
PEN & SWORD BOOKS LTD
47 Church Street, Barnsley, South Yorkshire, S70 2AS, England
E-mail: enquiries@pen-and-sword.co.uk
Website: www.pen-and-sword.co.uk
or
PEN & SWORD BOOKS
1950 Lawrence Rd, Havertown, PA 19083, USA
E-mail: uspen-and-sword@casematepublishers.com
Website: www.penandswordbooks.com

Contents

Foreword *by Ken Cunningham* vii
Introduction ix
  1. Microsurgery in Australia 1
  2. Consultant Surgeon at Stoke Mandeville Hospital 13
  3. Research 35
  4. Early Military Involvement 43
  5. Military Involvement as a Surgeon 51
  6. Medical Care in Disasters and Wars 65
  7. Motor Racing Track Doctor 105
  8. St John Ambulance 115
  9. Overseas Teaching, Work and Conferences 129
10. Teaching, Examining, Media and Medico-Legal Work 151
11. Patients 169
12. Honours and Awards 181
13. A View of the Changes in Health Care during the last
    Fifty Years 187
References 199
Index 201

Foreword

I was both surprised and honoured to be asked to write this Foreword for Anthony. Surprised, because a copy of *Who's Who* and a world atlas are recommended when reading his autobiography, and honoured because, as a hospital manager, clinicians and managers are not always natural colleagues. Having said that, Anthony is a friend and his enthusiasm to take on almost any clinical challenge is both endearing and uncommon in my experience. His surgical skills are in part a function of his engineering background as well as his extensive experience in treating all manner of conditions across every continent including Antarctica.

As you read this account of his life as a doctor and surgeon, the names of famous clinicians, celebrities and royalty are mentioned on every other page. His travels take us across continents to learn about people and customs as well as wildlife and particularly birds that we read about in *National Geographic*. Is he the Phileas Fogg of doctors?

What does come across is that this is a man of endless energy and endeavour who is determined to experience life to the full whilst helping injured patients to cope and recover from their injuries and burns. His work with the Bradford fire victims was a heroic effort and many patients owe their recovery to his skills and dedication.

An A&E consultant once told me that she got an adrenaline rush when she heard Ambulance 'blues and twos'. 'It's what I was trained for,' she told me. After Bradford, Anthony has travelled to war zones and disasters like a moth to a flame. His self-belief and determination that he can and does make a difference are exceptional qualities and doctors and clinical staff like him are a godsend to many impoverished and desperate people in less fortunate parts of the world. Many of the accounts of his involvement are harrowing and awe-inspiring. Being held up and robbed at gunpoint in Bosnia would have been enough to dissuade normal people from leaving these shores again but not Anthony! It's hard to estimate the impact he has had on burn care across the globe, and in teaching the military in the UK and several other countries, but it is clearly substantial.

Plastic Surgery in Wars, Disasters and Civilian Life

I know him from my ten years at Stoke Mandeville Hospital. There were two specialist centres included in a district general hospital: the Burn and Plastics Unit and the National Spinal Injuries Centre. One was based in wartime huts, the other in a custom-built modern centre. The care given to patients in both was second to none. I have no doubt that the outcomes in the outback of Australia or the native villages of South Africa where Anthony worked were just as successful as in any modern facility. It is the doctors, nurses and other clinical staff who make the difference and Anthony made sure that he always had an excellent team.

Clinical research should always aspire to improve the outcome or understanding of medical conditions. There is no doubt that the Burns Trust led by Anthony met these criteria. The money raised should always be trackable to the research. In my experience this is something that doesn't always happen in other areas of research.

It is difficult to read this book and not spare a thought for his wife Vivian, herself a distinguished GP. Her support and contribution to their lives has undoubtedly been a major factor in helping Anthony achieve many of the things he has. They are both excellent hosts and seem to find time for activities in the days that most of us would struggle to keep up with.

To describe Anthony as a doctor and surgeon is like saying Churchill was a politician. Both statements are true but completely miss the scale of the contribution they made. And yes, he did meet Churchill on one occasion!

Ken Cunningham

Introduction

Over the last few years several people with whom I have been talking have suggested that I should write down the story of my life. When that number reached about a hundred, I decided to have a go. Covid-19 with its lockdowns has given me time, and also a relief from total boredom.

I was the only child of a couple who divorced when I was 5 years old and was brought up by my mother as a sickly child with tuberculosis. After the war we lived in a two-bedroomed bungalow, half of which was let out to produce an income. Because of my illness, which had eventually been cured by daily injections of streptomycin for three months, I did not start at the local primary school until I was nearly 8 years old. When starting to write these memoirs I realised the major importance of the several scholarships that I was awarded, and particularly the first one that took me from that local primary school to Bancroft's School, a local public school.

My life since has been a mixture of work and research, both as an engineer and as a surgeon; of hobbies, particularly natural history and conservation; of sport; and of travels to more than a hundred countries, sometimes for pleasure, but more often for work or for natural history study.

One of my major problems has been the lack of a diary. Until the last few years I had always thought that I did not need one as I had an unusual, almost photographic, memory. Unfortunately that memory is now departing before this autobiography is not only not finished, but almost before it is starting. Luckily I have my passports, calendars and diaries over the years, and my wife Vivian has kept some records of our travels together over the last fifty years. I have been phoning and emailing friends for names and dates, for which my thanks, and the web has been incredibly useful. And I have also discovered that the worst thing about retirement is the loss of one's secretaries.

I had also not realised to the extent that I now do, that from about the age of 8 or 9 I have nearly always been involved in teaching. But there has also been a selection of other interests, in such things as cars and in reconstructing old houses.

Plastic Surgery in Wars, Disasters and Civilian Life

Long before I finished writing, and as the length of the text increased, I realised that my life would have to be split into three or four separate parts. Both I and other people think that the most important and interesting part has been my life as a consultant surgeon. That is the content of this book. My training and work as a chemical engineer, and then as a biochemical engineer, and the subsequent change to medicine have been described in another book.

After my change of career I started, as all doctors do, as a medical student. I returned to Cambridge and to my old College, St Catharine's. As I already had a degree I required only two years there instead of the normal three. After teaching and working in Zambia for the following summer I then moved to Worcester College, Oxford. Oxford was very unusual in that there were only twenty-six clinical medical students in my intake. Five of us had degrees in other subjects and there were three with PhDs. As well as the normal elective period of four months in South Africa, I also spent two months of the course in Michigan before my graduation.

Then followed my training as a surgeon and then as a plastic surgeon, which unusually included six months in southern Africa. This period of my life, which includes what was then a very important part of my life as a sportsman, is being published by Matador as *Scholarship Boy to Engineer, Plastic Surgeon and Sportsman*.

* * *

This book starts with my year in Australia learning microsurgery, which has relevance to both military and civilian injuries. I had already been appointed as a consultant plastic, hand and burn surgeon at Stoke Mandeville and other hospitals when the Bradford Football Stadium fire occurred in May 1985, in the aftermath of which I was very involved. As the years progressed I also became involved with the Spinal Injuries Unit, and with the work of various colleagues. Chapter 3 covers the research which still occupies me. Chapters 4 and 5 describe my work with both the British and the Egyptian military forces and with the United States Air Force.

The next part (Chapters 6 to 11) contains the unusual aspects of my professional career, including my work in six international disasters and four wars. I have also worked or taught in forty-five foreign countries and operated in twenty-five of them. It includes motor-racing doctoring

Foreword

and sixteen years with the Royal Protection Group, some of my most memorable patients, and my teaching, examining, legal and media work.

Chapter 12 is concerned with my awards, as somewhere along the way, as well as several scholarships, I collected an OBE and an OStJ, as well as the Fellowships of four national organisations. The final chapter consists of my comments on the changes in health care in the United Kingdom over the last fifty years, both the successes and the disasters.

If I live long enough, the third book, which is now nearly finished, will include my early life, my schooling and my family life, but this will be of more interest to my present and future family. The fourth book which has been started concerns my travels and work in conservation.

In these eighty-plus years I somehow found time to get married, and have remained so for fifty years, with two daughters and now four grandchildren.

Chapter 1

Microsurgery in Australia

I have started with this chapter as it was such an important part of my training, and was an essential part of my work for the next thirty years. After the offer of a year's Fellowship I had saved up a month of my leave and we set off from Yorkshire as a family to Australia in June 1981. It was extraordinarily lucky that at the time we had friends in the Philippines, in Malaysia and in Brunei, and we had organised to visit them all. These visits will be described in another book. The only medical aspect was a visit to the excellent hospital in Brunei. At the end of the day the superintendent showing me round said that I would be welcome to work there at any time, including now!

In Melbourne we had very long-time friends, Clive and Pat Minton. Clive had been my trainer when I qualified as a bird ringer four years previously. He had gone to Australia six months before us as the managing director of a major company. When we arrived in Melbourne they were away, but had very kindly arranged to lend us their house and car. We moved in, and the following day, 16 July, I went to the microsurgical laboratory which was part of St Vincent's Hospital close to the centre of the city. There I met Mr Bernard O'Brien, the founder and director of the unit. In standard Australian fashion his first comments were about the useless English cricket team then performing in Leeds. Three days later he regretted his comments when we won with the famous result, and I was able to get my own back – but he took it all in good humour. Never give in to the Ozzies!

St Vincent's was a Roman Catholic hospital in two main parts. There was the old public hospital and a much more recent private hospital. Most of the consultants were Catholic and many of the nurses were nuns. The two parts were adjacent to each other in Fitzroy, a poor area of Melbourne to the east of the city centre, and with a relatively high percentage of aboriginal people. It had been set up in 1893 by the Sisters of Charity. In 1899 William Moore, a surgeon working in the hospital, wrote a book called *Plastic Surgery*, the first book to be published in English on the subject. In the 1960s Dr Richard (Dick) Newing, who had trained as a general surgeon and then became involved in plastic surgery at Mount Vernon Hospital in England, had been appointed to set up a plastic surgery unit subsidiary to that of Sir Benjamin Rank at the Heidelberg Military Hospital and the Royal Melbourne Hospital. These hospitals had both treated war-injured Australians. As well as the injured, they also operated on head and neck cancers. I did clinics with Dick Newing, but he was not involved in microsurgery or head and neck surgery and I never saw him operate.

In 1965 Dr Bernard O'Brien had returned to a research post from his training in Oxford, Salisbury and New York. He had been inspired in New York by the microvascular work of Harold Buncke, and in a visit to Russia by microlymphatic surgery. A short time later he set up the Microsurgery Research Centre (later to be renamed The O'Brien Institute). From talking to his colleagues and reading about his life, it seems he was a quite remarkable man with the will to succeed born into him from his early years. At Melbourne University he had been the pole vault champion – and as pole vaulting had been my athletic specialty at school I was in sympathy. Throughout his life he had been awarded a variety of national and international honours, and also held positions, normally as President, of various societies and institutions. His early work at the hospital was developing microsurgical instruments, but his greatest success was setting up the microsurgical laboratory, and then persuading charities and the government to fund the research with four international microsurgery Fellowships. More than one hundred Fellows from twenty countries have been trained through these Fellowships. By 1981 his best years as a surgeon had passed, as retinitis pigmentosa meant that his peripheral vision was very poor and only working down a microscope was really possible for him. Much of his operating had in the recent past years been done by Wayne Morrison, and when I was there the Fellows did much of the operating. I remember during one operation I said, 'I am going to cut there.' 'Where?' he said and stuck his finger in front of my knife. I unfortunately just nicked his finger! 'I'll get you,' he said – but as it really was not my fault I was forgiven.

O'Brien intensely disliked his rival, Professor Ian Taylor at the Royal Melbourne Hospital, I think particularly as one of Bernard's juniors had borrowed some instruments from St Vincent's and taken them to the Royal Melbourne where Ian Taylor and the junior had done the world's first successful microvascular flap transfer. When I was there we were forbidden to go to the Royal Melbourne, or to talk to the people working there about our research. This was somewhat difficult for Vivian and myself, as a very good British friend, Clive Reed, was the Fellow there at the time. Although we did meet with Clive and his wife regularly, I honoured the situation by never discussing the research of either unit.

In the 1990s, never having smoked in his life, Bernard developed lung cancer, and died in 1993 at the young age of 69.

In 1972 Allan Mcleod joined the unit. He was an ex-RAAF surgeon and much of his work was at the renamed Heidelberg Repatriation Hospital, which had become involved in head and neck cancer treatment as well as working with war veterans. The Fellows did some work with him, and particularly when a microvascular flap was needed. Outside the hospital he was a water polo player, and also involved in the surf rescue teams. I never discovered why anyone wanted to swim around Victoria as the water was very cold. At least the sharks in the area were friendly.

In 1976 Wayne Morrison, who had trained in Glasgow, Paris and Miami, joined the unit as a specialist hand surgeon. He rapidly became involved in the microsurgery work and in the research. He was one of the most remarkable surgeons with whom I trained. One of my fellow Fellows was convinced that he had a parrot with X-ray eyes sitting on his shoulder and telling him where abnormal anatomy was situated. I never saw him make a mistake, and he had the other advantage to the patient, as well as to the staff, of being a rapid operator and a good teacher. In his youth he had been a champion boxer, winning his Blue at the University of Melbourne.

A year later the fifth consultant appointed was David Jenner, who had been trained in Norwich. He was a general plastic surgeon, and we only met on ward rounds for general discussions.

That was the clinical team when I was there, and they were augmented by an Australian registrar, Andrew Jenkins, with whom the Fellows shared the on-call cover.

We were given a basic Fellowship scholarship grant and were registered as medical practitioners in the state of Victoria for one year. In the 1980s all doctors in Australia were registered in only one state. The Fellows were appointed on a rolling basis, and when I was there they were Suman Das from America, Orthon Papadopoulos from Greece, Otto Weiglein from Canada, Hung-Chi Chen from Taiwan and Vaughan Bowen, an Englishman who came from, and returned to, Canada.

Both of the St Vincent's Hospitals did a range of plastic surgery, with specialisation in microsurgery and hand surgery. The system was very different from the United Kingdom as the majority of patients were medically insured, which was a government requirement for anybody who was employed. The result of this was that a patient coming in in the middle of the night with a small laceration, which in England would have been sutured by the junior trainee on call, was sutured by a consultant to earn a fee. The registrar therefore had very little operating experience except assisting, and operated himself only on the relatively rare uninsured patient. I know that Andrew Jenkins, the registrar at the time, was not very happy about this. The consultant's income was dependent on the insurance payments as they did not receive a salary from the hospital unless they were rare full-time employees. The other factor which affected the income of qualified surgeons was the number of them in existence. In the state of Victoria there were about eighty plastic surgeons, compared with a hundred in the whole of the United Kingdom, and that was why a hospital attachment was so important. One consultant told me that for the first five years after setting up his practice he would not go away even for a weekend in case he missed a referral. After five years he had enough of a referral pattern to afford a week away! Another difference between Melbourne and England, which caused me some confusion when I arrived, was that in Australia some surgeons were known as 'Doctor' and some as 'Mister'. In England all qualified surgeons are called 'Mister' for historical reasons. They were the unqualified barbers and the bone-setters, and the physicians who were called 'Doctor' would not let them use the title. When surgeons became fully medically qualified, they decided to retain the title of 'Mister', which we now consider an honour.

The programme was such that I would spend the first few weeks in the animal laboratory learning and practising the basic microsurgical techniques, and would then assist at operations as well as starting research projects. If I proved satisfactory, I would then on occasions lead the team in operations, and particularly the acute replantations. There would also be opportunities to earn some money to add to my basic Fellowship by assisting the local surgeons with their private practice.

My first port of call when I arrived therefore was to a scrappy entrance in a back street between the hospitals. Inside was a far from scrappy laboratory run by an excellent old-time sister, Maris Williams. I had learned many years before that the first and most important thing to do in a laboratory is to make friends with the boss. Maris was a farmer's daughter, and we would spend happy hours talking about the natural history of the area. I would list the species and numbers of the snakes and other animals that I had seen the previous weekend, and she would fill in with information about them. And all to the disbelief of the other people in the laboratory, many of whom, despite being Australian born, had never or rarely seen a snake, and certainly not a platypus in the wild. There were two assistants who were our technical teachers, and two local research assistants. I was lucky to be adopted by Sue McKay, who was lovely, gentle and an excellent teacher. The other assistant was Liz Wilson. I had much less to do with her, but my memory tells of some excellent parties at her parents' house. Within a few weeks Sue had taught me how to do both microvascular and microlymphatic anastomoses. There were also two research assistants, Geraldine Nightingale and a lass of Italian origin. The animal house was in the yard behind the lab, and was run by separate staff. The rules for animal experimentation in Australia were very much more sensible than those in England, and the anti-vivisection movement far less vocal. In overall control was a qualified veterinary surgeon who had to approve the research, and the conditions in which the animals were kept and cared for. Later in the year this was very useful to me, particularly when it was combined with the agreement amongst all vets that they would treat any injured native animal without charging. Just up from my house I had found a tawny frogmouth, a large uncommon nocturnal bird with sharp claws and a very sharp and powerful beak. It had a damaged and clearly infected eye. I managed to get it into a box and took it to the lab to discuss the treatment with the vet. It is known that in all animals, including humans, the reaction from one damaged eye can spread to the other eye. The vet and I agreed that the only possible treatment which might preserve the bird was for the injured eye to be removed. Into the lab we went. He anaesthetised the bird, and I removed the eye and repaired the socket. After the operation the bird stayed in the animal house for a few days, its health improving rapidly, and then I took it back and released it in the field where I had found it. It flew happily away.

The animals that we were using in the laboratory were mainly rabbits and greyhounds. The latter were donated to the unit, because either they were too old to race, or they had been failures on the track. After the surgery the anaesthetic was changed to cause their death, and no pain would have been felt at any time.

Whilst I was in the laboratory phase, discussions about a research programme started. In Australia there was a major problem, particularly in ladies who had had radiotherapy for breast cancer, of a very swollen (lymphodaemic) arm afterwards. Bernie O'Brien had considered that doing lymphovenous anastomoses after the radiotherapy would reduce this swelling. It was a difficult research problem because very few of the ladies had previously had the standard compression treatment of the arm on a daily basis, and their arms were markedly enlarged and perhaps weighing two to three times the normal, causing a major loss of function.

At the time Vaughan Bowen had just started in the laboratory and his opinion was that the research suggested for him was not possible because the vessels that he was expected to anastomose were too small. They were actually about 1.5mm external diameter. At the time I was practising lymphovenous anastomoses in the laboratory. This was on vessels approximately 0.75mm external diameter. Susan McKay brought Vaughan over so that he could see the size of the vessels I was working on. He became thoughtful, and then said he would try again.

I was doing the relevant clinical work on the patients with Hung-Chi Chen. One problem was that the compression treatment was started after we had operated on a patient, and this made comparison with the untreated arm difficult. The basic results showed that if there had been a long-term problem, the gain was minimal. What clearly worked, however, was performing the operation soon after the radiotherapy, which reduced the potential swelling of the arm. The work was jointly published.

The other project in which I became involved was looking at the role of anticoagulant drugs on the success of arterial anastomoses, particularly if the vessels were damaged. I did this with the help of a cardiologist at the Austin Hospital, Dr Jim Angus. Towards the end of my time this was going well and would have been suitable for writing up for a higher degree. Unfortunately a critical part of the apparatus that I was using broke down, and it was not replaceable for several months. When I returned to Bradford I carried on the research with Sonia Bannerjee and then Andrew Wilmshurst. This was successfully submitted for a higher degree.

What made the unit successful was the number of patients requiring microsurgery. This was exaggerated because at the time, with the exception of some work at the Royal Melbourne, there were no other units in Australia doing microsurgical work. The average weekly caseload was two cold (waiting list) patients and one acute replant or revascularisation.

After the time in the lab, one or more of the Fellows would be the assistant(s), normally to Wayne as the principal surgeon. Promotion up the line of usefulness depended on one's ability and experience. Bernie would often be in the theatre, but rarely scrubbed up. I well remember one case of a finger replant operation. It was a difficult case as the finger had been pulled off, rather than cut off. The first anastomosis failed, and from Bernie in the corner came the command, 'Do it again.' It was redone, and, not surprisingly to us, it failed again. 'Do it again' came from the corner. We thought that we were really wasting our time, but we did it again and it worked! This was a very valuable lesson for us all.

The acute cases could come in at any time of the day or the night. What could be replanted? – fingers (either one or several), thumbs and ears – though I never saw a successful case of the latter in Melbourne or in the rest of my career. And we had a single case of a penis which the patient, having cut it off, then decided he would like put back. It was an interesting and successful challenge. If the part to be replanted was cooled when the accident had happened, then there were 8 to 12 hours available for the operation. The more urgent cases were when a digit or part of the hand or foot had had the blood vessels cut, but was still attached. This could not then be satisfactorily cooled, and the time limit rapidly dropped to about 4 hours.

I remember three acute cases. The first was an elderly Chinese gentleman who had cut off half of one finger. Normally we would recommend that the stump be refashioned. However, this gentleman had a belief that he had to die 'whole', and would we please try to replant it. We did try, but unfortunately unsuccessfully.

The second case was towards the end of my year. Late one afternoon one theatre was occupied by a cold case when an acute case came in. She was a young girl needing a single finger replant. I was asked to do this on my own in the second theatre, and 2½ hours later the replant was successfully finished.

The third case was incredible. A 14-year-old girl had caught her long hair in the back of a tractor. The machinery had pulled off the whole of her scalp, including her forehead and an ear, with skin down to her neck on that side. The accident had occurred several hundred miles away in the north of Victoria. The part was cooled, and she was flown down to St Vincent's. The replant required two consultants, Allan McLeod and Wayne Morrison, and two Fellows working 2-hour shifts. Some 24 hours later, and twenty-four units of blood later, it was all replanted. The problem was not the microsurgery, but stopping the bleeding from the scalp without damaging the blood supply. A very small part of the neck skin died and needed a small correction a few days later. Without the replant her appearance for the rest of her life would have been horrific, and similar to some of the worst burn cases. In fact, we heard that her occupation some years later was as a model. (*see* Plates 1.1 to 1.3.)

The waiting list cases were split between microvascular flaps and microlymphatic work for post-radiotherapy ladies. The latter were a test of our skill at anastomosing very small vessels. The only microvascular case that I saw with similar size vessels was transplanting one of two intra-abdominal testes in a very small boy to its correct place in the scrotum. This was done when the boy was 2 years old before he became infertile for life.

Another waiting list patient I remember very well was a 6ft 8in tall man who came to us from Sydney with a bone cancer of his lower leg. He had refused amputation of that leg, which would have been the standard treatment. The only possible alternative was to use the fibula from the other leg as a bone transplant. He came to us with his senior orthopaedic surgeon, who at that time was not licensed to practise in Victoria. I had been asked to scrub up to protect the vessels that we were going to be needed for the transplant, whilst a local consultant orthopaedic surgeon excised the tibia bone in which the tumour was growing. I was having some problems protecting the vessels when an arm from the Sydney surgeon appeared, took the scalpel from the local surgeon and passed it to me, with the comment, 'I think that looks easier from your side.' The local orthopaedic surgeon walked out, and I finished the tumour excision. The fibula from the other leg was made ready, and I was preparing the vessels that were to be used in the leg into which it was going. The standard procedure is to clamp an artery before cutting it, and then to test the flow. At the time I was operating down the microscope, and as I released the clamp, I said, 'That looks a reasonable flow.' The Sydney surgeon muttered, 'That is what I call English understatement.' When I looked round the blood flow had hit him squarely in the face! All went well with the operation, and it is possible that this was the first time that such an operation had been performed anywhere in the world, and certainly the transplanted fibula was the longest anywhere. I heard later that the patient did manage to walk afterwards.

My experience and skill built up over the year and the research was going well until the instrument failure. I had no involvement with medical students, but at one time Wayne asked me to assist with a mock examination for the Fellowship of the Royal Australian College of Surgeons that he was running. There was a section on the treatment of burns, of which Wayne had had almost no experience in his particular training. This was very much my subject, and as I was doing the viva examination with the students, I could see Wayne making copious notes. He told me later that he used the notes when he was the examiner at the actual exam.

I was given the month of January as my holiday. By this time we had bought a Volkswagen camper van, and Vivian and I and our two girls had decided to travel north as far as possible, and also to visit friends of mine in Sydney and distant relations of hers outside Brisbane on the way back.

In 1981 there was no dual carriageway joining the two largest cities in the country, and north of Sydney the road up to Cairns was often single track across bridges where vehicles going north had the right of way. Four days later we arrived in Cairns. I had been advised to drop into the Flying Doctor base and introduce myself. I was immediately asked if I would like to fly up to the far north and help in some of the clinics. They did not appear to worry that I was not registered in Queensland as I would be regarded as a visitor. The Australian Flying Doctor Service is a charity that started in 1928 in Queensland. I believe that it was originally started so that farm workers could call for advice, and be taken by air to hospital when needed. It has since spread to also providing the same service for Aboriginal communities. The service at Cairns covered the communities in the Cape York Peninsula in north Queensland, and also the mines, mainly bauxite, in the area. In 1982 the government rules were that the only people allowed to visit these communities were medical, teaching and management personnel. I was introduced to the doctor who would be going. He had recently qualified from Queensland University, and, as he had been on a scholarship, he had to work for the government for two years as a payback.

I left Vivian to entertain our two daughters by the pool, and I, the doctor, a nurse and a logistics officer met the lady pilot early the next morning at the airport and flew north to Cooktown on the east coast. There we contacted the resident nurse and assistant and did an out-patient clinic. It was remarkably similar to the clinics that I had done in Africa. Some 60–70 per cent of the patients had a venereal disease, and some had bad chests or small infected wounds, but I do not remember a single patient with a major problem. We then flew to Weipa on the west side of the peninsula, and did a similar clinic. The next day we drove south in a Land Cruiser to an Aboriginal community and did another clinic. I then arranged for a local man to take me for a natural history walk. This was fascinating, especially seeing all the uses of the vegetation. I was fed a small passion fruit, which was excellent, and several other berries that I did not recognise. I was also shown the leaves of a sandpaper tree. Their upper surface is sufficiently rough to act as sandpaper when tools and weapons are being made. Luckily my guide failed to find a witchetty grub as I would have had to eat it raw or lose face.

We then drove further south to a second community, which in itself was interesting in that alcohol, which can be a major problem with the people, was totally banned by the community and anyone found drinking was thrown out. The amazing fact was that we were greeted with broad Scottish accents. It turned out that a Scottish Christian charity had been based in the area since before the war. The story was related that during the war an American plane was flying from Cairns to Papua New Guinea. The pilot had been told to follow the coastline, and when the coastline turned left to carry on to the north. Unfortunately, he failed to follow the order and the plane ended up flying south instead of north until it ran out of fuel. The crew had to ditch the plane in the very shallow Gulf of Carpentaria. As they got out of the plane they noticed a row of local tribesmen, with spears in their right hands, standing along the shore. Not knowing what to do next, the crew climbed onto the top of the plane and the two sides regarded each other. Some hour or so later the tribesmen called out in their marked Scottish accent, 'When you have sat long enough, would ye like a coup o char?'

Before we left we were also shown a crocodile farm, which raised money for the community.

We drove back in worsening weather to Weipa, and there discovered that a teenage lad from the Torres Islands to the north had come into the hospital with severe abdominal pain. On examination he clearly had a classical appendicitis, which needed surgery. The pilot then told us that the weather was not suitable for flying. The doctor and I looked at each other. There was an operating theatre and equipment in the small base hospital. The anaesthetic machine had apparently not been serviced for some years but appeared to be complete, and the necessary gases were present. The next problem was that the doctor had never removed an appendix. We agreed that he would anaesthetise the boy with my help, I would then do the operation, and he would sign the notes. We were just about to put the boy to sleep when the pilot appeared, saying 'The weather has improved, and I can now fly.' What would have been my last appendicectomy thus did not happen, and we all flew back to Cairns. It had proved to be an interesting three days.

We had a further two days in Cairns as a family and then meandered slowly south. I had a bird contact near Tully, one of the wettest places on earth, whom we had arranged to visit. He was doing a PhD thesis on golden bower birds. After him and his wife, I was the third non-indigenous person in the world to see the nests of this species.

I nearly had to do some medical work when a motor-cyclist coming up the hill crashed. Unfortunately he was dead when we got to him. I did have to remove a multitude of small leeches from us all, including one that had got behind a lower eyelid. It had luckily not attached itself, and there was no bleeding after its removal. After a very interesting month, it was back to Melbourne for five months.

The work for me was fascinating. Vivian was also registered as a doctor for the year and was much sought after to do GP locums. She was not impressed with the Australian system when compared to the British system. Any patient could see any doctor, and there was no centralised note system. She could ask why a patient had a scar on their abdomen, and the patient would say that they had had an operation but did not know what had been found or done. She was also asked to take totally unnecessary weekly blood pressure readings on patients who were not insured, as the government would pay the doctor. I understand that much of this has now changed after some court cases.

On the social side, whilst we were staying in the Mintons' house for two weeks we had found a house to rent in Eaglemont, about 1½ miles from the hospital. Settling into the house was made more difficult as we had sent our two large trunks by sea. Unfortunately the dock workers were on strike and therefore all our warm clothes, our ski equipment and the useful things that we needed in the house all sat on the docks for six weeks whilst we froze in the house that had, as was common in Australia, no central heating. One evening I damaged my back for the only time in my life having a judo fight with my wife Vivian to warm up, and then spent the next few weeks sleeping at night on a mattress on the floor. We enrolled the children into the Methodist Ladies College. This was in itself interesting as Tasha, our younger daughter, then aged 5, had already been at school in England but was too young to attend school in Australia. They solved this by promoting her to the class above her age. I bought the VW camper van and equipped it for the four of us to be able to stay in it.

Within the department the social life was brilliant, and far better than in any other job that I had done – or would do in the future. On our first weekend we were welcomed to a 'Barbie' to meet the department and their partners. The fact that it was cold and raining deterred no one. Throughout our stay similar events and dinners were held regularly, perhaps to say farewell to old Fellows or welcome new ones, or for any suitable excuse. One day Bernie asked me to drive him in his new Jaguar to the Melbourne Cricket Ground, where I saw my one and only Australian Rules football match. Whilst we were in Australia both Vivian and I became addicted to Australian wines, which could be bought in litre boxes. Through the Mintons I made contacts with the local bird ringers (called banders in Australia, as they are in America), and every weekend when not on call we were banding shorebirds at Werribee sewage works, or forest birds at Toolangi with Richard Loyn, or travelling in the Grampians or other areas of the countryside. At one of our parties Richard met our research assistant, who despite being born in Melbourne and having lived her 30-plus years there, had never driven off a tarred road, or really been into the countryside. Richard rapidly changed all that.

Then the time came to return home. We arranged to travel via New Zealand, where Vivian had a relative, and then via California, where we stayed with a plastic surgeon colleague, Sam Wong, and his wife. I had trained with Sam at the Birmingham Accident Hospital. Arriving back in Leeds we discovered that the person who had rented our house had left it, and the garden, in a terrible state, and had not paid the rent for several months. After a major clean-up we moved back in.

It was a marvellous and unforgettable year, although even with the Fellowship, a scholarship from the British Association of Plastic Surgeons and Vivian's income, because of the school fees and the house problems we were £5,000 poorer, but much richer in experience.

Chapter 2

Consultant Surgeon at Stoke Mandeville Hospital

Towards the end of my time in Australia a permanent job was coming up at St Vincent's Hospital, which was half research and half clinical. This was an ideal combination for me, and I would very much have enjoyed the challenge. I made some basic enquiries but was firmly told that they had an Australian, Julian Pribaz, lined up for the job. He was somebody I had not met, because he was at that stage in America obtaining specialised training. He came back to the job some two years later but, unfortunately for the unit in Melbourne, he only stayed for three or four years before he up-stumped and returned to America. Ever since then they have said that they should have had me. By that time, of course, I had my consultant post in England and Vivian's general practice was all arranged.

The advertisement for the post at Stoke Mandeville Hospital appeared. I had never visited the hospital and knew very little about it. I went along to look around the hospital, and to meet the two consultants, Mr Bailey and Mr Desai. In many ways it was an ideal job for me in that it combined the Directorship of the Burn Unit with hand surgery. It was also agreed that if I were to be appointed, I would have one day a week to do research. In those days it was normal to meet, on the evening prior to the interview, the various members of the rest of the hospital at a sherry party. Wives were also invited. This I might say has totally and utterly changed now and would be considered 'Very Bad Form'. The day after the sherry party, my interview went well. There were two other candidates who had worked at the hospital in the past, and also Richard Matthews and Tony Atwood, and these were obviously strong competition. It was normal to have a lay chairperson for any consultant interview committee, and on this occasion it was Mrs Gillian Miscampbell. She had not asked any questions throughout the interview, but at the end she said to me, 'Having listened to your answers during the interview, and having read your curriculum vitae, how would you react if I said you would appear to me to be somewhat eccentric?' My instant reply was, 'I would be flattered.' A chuckle went round the panel, and that was the end of the interview. After a short debate by the committee, I was appointed.

The next day I gave my notice to the Yorkshire board, knowing that I had three months to finish working there, to sell our house, to find a new home and schools for our daughters, and for Vivian to resign from her practice and find a new GP post. And during that three months occurred the tragedy that was the Bradford Football Club fire (*see* Chapter 6) which, together with my new post, was to revolutionise my future life.

Our house in Leeds was put on the market, and almost the first person who came round to view it bought it. Looking for a house in Buckinghamshire was more difficult. Firstly it was a long way to travel for viewings, and secondly an equivalent house there was far more expensive than in Leeds at that time. We looked at a variety of houses, having decided that we needed four bedrooms and ideally some grounds. We eventually came across Longmoor Farm in Aston Abbotts, about 6 miles from Stoke Mandeville. This was an early Victorian house, very much a working farm, and clearly in need of considerable restoration and updating. It had a covered courtyard in terrible condition in which animals and farm equipment were being kept. It was owned by Mr and Mrs Bellingham. Mr Bellingham was in fact Squadron Leader Don Bellingham, a renowned and highly decorated RAF bomber pilot from the Second World War. In conversation he once compared sitting on a combine harvester to flying a bomber, and said that was why he was a farmer. One of their daughters was Lynda Bellingham, a well known actress. We made an offer, with considerable help from the bank, and this was accepted, but unfortunately we could only afford 1½ acres of the land that was for sale. I do remember on one occasion when we were driving for a weekend to Buckinghamshire coming across an enormous amount of snow on each side of the road in the north of the county. Having come from Yorkshire, where one expected snow, this was somewhat of a nasty surprise as we had assumed that we were moving to the sunny south.

We found places for Clare and Natasha, our two daughters, at Maltman's Green Preparatory School, where they were to be weekly boarders. Vivian joined Dr Allan Machlachlan in the local general practice in Whitchurch, and I started my new job in the hospital in July 1985.

Stoke Mandeville was, and still is, an unusual hospital (*see* Plate 2.1). It originated in the 1830s when a cholera epidemic swept the country and more than fifty people in Aylesbury died. An isolation hospital was built in the 1890s and this developed into a 'fever' hospital, treating all forms of infectious diseases; a new 'isolation' hospital was added in 1933. (In fact my wife Vivian was a patient there with scarlet fever as a young child.) In 1939 the adjoining 90 acres were acquired by the War Office as the site for a new Emergency Services Hospital, and a new and enlarged hospital was created. This was made up of what were then modern one-storey Nissan huts with large gaps between each hut, and in each of these gaps was an underground bomb shelter. At that stage it was a District General Hospital looking after war-injured patients as well as patients from Aylesbury and the surrounding area. Then in 1941 a burn and plastic surgery unit was added by Mr Pomfret Kilner. He later became the Nuffield Professor of Plastic Surgery in Oxford in 1944, and was the only professor of plastic surgery for many years in the United Kingdom. The next major addition was the spinal injuries unit, created by Sir Ludwig Gutman in 1944. When I arrived in 1985 the plastic and burn unit had 80 beds and the spinal injury unit had 120 beds. It was therefore a small district general hospital with two world-famous units added to it. This did not always make relationships within the hospital easy.

My role as consultant also included doing out-patient clinics in the Battle Hospital, Reading, and in the Northampton General Hospital. I was given the role of Director of the Oxford Regional Burn Unit, one session a week to do research, and one session free which could be used for private practice. My appointment was a new post and did not follow a retirement. I made the seventh doctor in the department, with two other consultants, a senior registrar, a registrar and two senior house officers. There were no house surgeons. My two senior colleagues had both been there for several years.

Mr Bruce Bailey was a remarkable man. He had been an army surgeon and was also very involved in mountaineering. He was also one of the first surgeons in the world to do microvascular surgery, and in England was fêted in all the national papers for having successfully reconnected an agricultural worker's severed arm. He had also originated and developed the technique of repairing cleft lips within 24 hours of birth. He had been Director of the Oxford Regional Burn Unit for many years, and passed this post to me when I started. We shared the large hand surgery workload. Tragically in his fifties he developed Parkinson's disease which necessitated his early retirement. He then developed a malignant melanoma on his back which caused his death in 2001.

My other colleague was Mr Sanu Desai. Sanu had initially qualified in India and then emigrated to England for his plastic surgery training, which included a period of instruction under Mr Tom Barclay in Bradford, who described him to me as an excellent surgeon. Sanu took over and developed the early cleft repair work with the orthodontist Mr Brian Christie, and was appointed a Royal College of Surgeons Hunterian Professor for this work. He also edited the book *Neonatal Surgery of the Cleft Lip and Palate* in 1997. We shared the hypospadias repairs and breast surgery for reconstruction after cancer, and breast reductions. He was not involved in hand surgery or the burn unit.

My initial working practice was therefore laid down when I started, and it was the perfect combination for the interests that I had developed during my training. Within the department I covered the burn unit at all times, and when I was on leave or working elsewhere the senior registrar would do the cover with Bruce as the back-up. We were all involved in the skin cancers and the breast reconstructions. The on-call load now sounds horrific, but it was eased by having extremely experienced registrars. Vivian's on-call commitments with her general practice and police surgeon's work, to which she could be called at almost any time, were similarly demanding. It was eased somewhat as our daughters were at boarding school and during termtime at least did not need ferrying around.

The workload changed a little over the years. One major change occurred after I had done a microvascular transfer of nerves and a muscle into the face of a patient who had total paralysis on one side from a malignant parotid tumour some years previously. This worked well and Mr Martin Mace, a maxillo-facial surgeon, began to send me more of his patients. He then asked if I would do all of the parotid surgeries. This was a new and very challenging field. The majority of parotid tumours are benign, but surgery is essential as malignant change can occur with time. Very careful excision is required in order to avoid damage to the facial nerve, and with Dr Richard Bunsell, the anaesthetist, we worked out the best way to do this. I finished up doing twenty or thirty parotid operations a year, without damaging a facial nerve (except intentionally in malignant cases). There was always that worrying time on the ward-round the day after the operation when you asked the patient to smile. There were some peculiar responses from the patient to the request, but always delight from me when the face moved equally on both sides.

In malignant parotid tumours one of the more obvious signs is the reduction in, or loss of, function of the facial nerve on that side of the face.

I developed the technique of biopsying the remaining facial nerve as it came out of the skull whilst the patient was still on the table, and, if it was clear of tumour on immediate analysis in the laboratory, putting in a nerve graft from a leg during the same operation. Nerves grow at about an inch a month and a few weeks later some function appeared in the facial muscles that were still alive. This saved a later two-stage operation with variable results and occasional failures. I only had three of these cases and regrettably did not publish the results.

Changes of staff did alter the pattern of my work to some extent, but of more significance were the junior surgeons. Plastic surgery as a specialty was spoilt for choice. It was the most popular of all the specialities, and not only in surgery. This meant that by the time a person became a registrar, and certainly a senior registrar, the competition had removed almost everybody who was not excellent. As time went by, this effect became less obvious as, to align with the EU working hours directive and the new training format, competition for promotion, and thereby the weeding out of less talented people, sadly decreased. Remembering the senior and the junior colleagues of those days has brought back many memories – nearly all of them good. Mr Padraic Regan, for example, who had been one of our SHOs, came back as a Senior Registrar and then as a Consultant in 1993. Both he and his wife, a dermatologist, were Irish, and the call to return home proved irresistible when a post was advertised in Galway. Padraic applied and was appointed there in 1997.

When Bruce retired in the late 1990s, he was replaced by Mr Tony Heywood, who took over half of the hand surgery. A new consultant, Mr Mark Scott, was appointed at about the same time and his special interest was breast surgery, in which he took on the major load and was excellent. Very sadly, although unbelievably fit and still a world champion in sky diving, and also having played cricket for one of the West Indian islands, he developed aggressive diabetes when in his late thirties. Knowing that he could lose his sight, at least to the extent of having to give up surgery, he decided to become a full-time private cosmetic surgeon in order to make enough money to enable him to retire early if it became necessary.

There were two further juniors who returned as consultants. Peter Budny was already a registrar in orthopaedic surgery when he came to Stoke Mandeville as an SHO to see some hand surgery. He enjoyed it so much that he converted to plastic surgery, and after his registrar and senior registrar training came back to us as a consultant. Mike Tyler was our second research fellow. He had already had an interesting year in Ljubljana in the clinic of Marko Gordina, a very well known reconstructive hand surgeon. Marko was tragically killed in a car crash in 1986. After completing his training, Mike came back to us as a consultant and has now taken on the chairmanship of the research trust (*see* Chapter 3).

The other senior registrars included Fiona Baillie, who became a consultant in Nottingham. When she arrived there, she went to her local bank to arrange a mortgage – and subsequently married the bank manager.

John Dickinson was an SHO when I arrived and already a very good surgeon, and was then promoted through the ranks to registrar and senior registrar. He was probably the last person to train completely within one unit. He became a consultant at Wexham Park Hospital. Another was Nick James. He was appointed as a consultant at the Lister Hospital, Stevenage. He was also involved as a motor-racing doctor at Silverstone.

I also remember another SHO who was training as a dermatologist. He had the good sense to come to us for special experience as a large part of the work of a dermatologist is minor surgery. Dr Andrew Tudway was the histopathologist with whom we were in closest contact. He always said that when a specimen in a bottle came to him, he could tell who had sent it just by looking at it. If it was in several pieces it was either from a GP or from a dermatologist. If it was in one piece, but with no margins around the tumour, it came from a general surgeon, but a good specimen with appropriate margins was from a plastic surgeon. At least the dermatologist, after his six months with us, would not fall into the first category!

In my sixteen years at Stoke Mandeville there would have been about a hundred juniors within the unit. They are commemorated in a row of photographs on the wall at the hospital. Some of them are memorable for a variety of reasons, but many are just distant memories. At least eighteen of them went on to become consultant plastic surgeons in three different countries.

On a regular basis there were also visiting surgeons from the British military, and from Egypt, South Africa, Greece and Turkey. These often came for a few weeks or several months whilst they were looking for a permanent post.

Burn Care and the Burn Unit

In the United Kingdom for the past century there has been a constant decline in the numbers of burn injuries, hospital admissions and deaths. The decline has been both in domestic and in industrial burns. This has been partly because of education, but much more because of changes in house heating and in electrical safety. An indication of the severity of the problem is that in the United Kingdom in the year 2000 there were about 175,000 people with a burn injury who attended an accident and emergency department; of these 13,000 were admitted to a hospital, and 300 people died.

As well as the causes of burn injuries there have also been major changes both in the facilities for care and in the treatment of burns. Specialised burn units were created, the world's first being established in Edinburgh in the 1930s by Mr A.B. Wallace. The idea was slowly spreading, and our unit was opened in 1956 when specialised burn units were still rare.

In 1985, when I took over the Stoke Mandeville unit, there was a unit in each of the thirteen NHS regions. As the Oxford Regional Unit we officially took all the burn patients who needed inpatient care from Oxfordshire, Buckinghamshire and Northamptonshire. Bed shortages elsewhere meant we also took patients from London and as far north as Birmingham.

In the last century the treatment of the burned patient had changed markedly. Before the Second World War the severely burned patient was put in a side room to die because of loss of fluid in the early stages or of infection if they survived the fluid loss. If they survived for the first few weeks the area of healing tissue was skin grafted. Major changes occurred during the war, when firstly the use of intravenous fluids and blood transfusions became common practice, and then with the introduction of antibiotics towards the end of the war.

The next major change came in the 1980s with the introduction of early surgery. The theory was that the area of skin that was burned was sterilised by the burn, and if surgery could be completed before infection set in, the patient had a much higher chance of survival. There were secondary gains in that the hospital in-patient time was reduced, and later scar correction and contracture surgery was also minimised. Early surgery required more theatre time, more blood and greater skill. The idea spread slowly even in developed countries and had not been introduced at Stoke Mandeville when I took over.

I immediately changed the unit to early surgery, and also introduced the various methods of reducing cross-infection that I had learned in Birmingham. There was surprisingly almost no resistance from the nursing staff, and as the early results became clear there was a rapid and complete acceptance. Over my years there these changes resulted in a reduction of the average hospital stay from twenty-three days to fewer than ten, and it also more than halved secondary reconstructive surgery. (This latter claim is an estimate as regrettably I did not research and publish accurate figures.)

The unit was housed in one of the temporary buildings put up during the Second World War and still being used. Ward 7X had four isolation cubicles for adults or children, and for adults there were also a three-bed ward and a four-bed ward. Children who did not need isolation went to the paediatric surgical ward, Ward 7, where there were available as many beds as were needed. The hospital intensive care unit had two isolation cubicles for our use. Unfortunately, if more were needed, we had to transfer the patient(s) to another burn unit. We had an unusual if not unique relationship with the ITU in that the patients were still under my care and Dr Richard Bunsell, the Director, and his team were responsible for the airway only. In other hospitals the overall care of the patient was transferred to the ITU consultants, which was not always satisfactory as their juniors in particular would have had very little burn experience.

Many of the ward staff had been there for several years and were vastly experienced and excellent. I was extremely lucky and grateful that both I and my reforms were accepted straightaway. The senior sister was Miss Diana Horn and the other sister was Mrs Susan Fox. On her retirement Diana was replaced by Mrs Adele Jones. Amongst the senior nurses were Mrs Nancy Simmonds and Mrs Jan Cooke. Other staff whom I remember were Bea Cameron and Gail Miller. The nursing of burn patients is an extremely demanding job, both for the skills needed in doing the dressings but also psychologically. The first problem is the deaths. It is possible to work out the chances of a patient dying based on their age, the extent of their burns, whether there was damage to their breathing through inhalation of hot gases, and also whether they had other injuries to make the situation worse. If a patient is certain to die, then the kindest thing is to treat them with painkillers, a cup of tea and a nurse or a family member to talk to as they lose consciousness within a few hours and die peacefully. It would be possible to keep some of these patients alive for some days, but the outcome is inevitable, and the steps needed to prolong life are painful for the patient and for everybody looking after them. An early decision to allow a peaceful death has much to recommend it. The nurses completely agreed with me that the kindest and most appropriate treatment was to make the patient comfortable. There was a secondary part to this in that the estimate of burn area by inexperienced people was, and still is, notoriously poor. We always said that it was often overestimated by a factor of two, and if it came from one particular local hospital then three was the more likely factor. As the probable outcome was dependent on this estimation, we had a rule that all major burn patients were to be sent to us for a final assessment before the most appropriate treatment was decided. So again, this put added stress on the nurses. In my experience, however, the greatest upset came when we had been working hard to keep a patient alive for some weeks but they died. These patients had often become friends as well as a medical challenge.

Burn surgery requires a large team and often requires a warm theatre. This is especially true when the patients are children (*see* Plate 2.2). Much of the success of the unit was down to the superb anaesthetic care given by Dr Bunsell. By chance we had both done some of our training at the Birmingham Accident Hospital, and his skill as an anaesthetist was paramount. (In future chapters I shall describe his work with me in Bosnia and Azerbaijan.)

Help is always needed in a burn unit from a psychiatrist and from social workers, both for the patients and the staff. We always said that half of the patients had a psychiatric problem on admission, and 100 per cent of them on discharge. When I started there was poor psychiatric cover but some months later a new psychiatric appointment was made by the hospital. Even before he had a chance to settle in, I recruited him to help with the unit. Dr Ian Wood was a remarkable person and excellent with the problems that often occurred in burn patients. He was a South African whose first degree in South Africa was in law. He then went to the United States on a Fulbright Scholarship to do a degree in economics, and finally to Oxford as a Rhodes Scholar to study medicine. His year at Oxford included Bill Clinton as another Rhodes scholar. Ian got first class honours in all his degrees and was also an outstanding sportsman who had represented South Africa at junior international level. Clearly he was a mixed-up kid – the ideal type for a psychiatrist.

In comparison to the early lack of psychiatric care, the social worker, Mrs Alison Hill, was exceptional. She covered all of the patients independently of their county of residence, and I was extremely grateful to her for the service that she provided. We were all very sad when some four years later she retired. And then disaster. Despite my protestations, it was decided that social workers would only look after patients (or clients, as they called them) from their own county. This meant that Buckinghamshire patients had some cover, and the other patients virtually nil. And none of the new social workers had anywhere near the experience of Alison. One was a total disaster. She returned to the parents an intentionally injured child, who was then readmitted a few days later with further and more severe injuries. In court both the police and I tried to have the social worker dismissed, but she was given another chance. After that, in emergency situations, I dealt with the police from whom I had an excellent service.

The other members of staff who were very important were the occupational therapist (Miss Maria Clark, who was in post both when I started and when I finished), the physiotherapist and the dietician. The latter two roles changed personnel more often.

The final essential people were the anaesthetist, normally Richard Bunsell, and the microbiologist, Dr Paul Gillett. By chance all three of us had trained at the Birmingham Accident Hospital, but not concurrently. At one time MRSA was a particularly nasty bug and could be spread between patients. Paul did a survey of all the wards in the hospital, and presented his findings at a lunchtime clinical meeting. Everyone in the hospital knew about nasty infected burns, and when the result was announced that the burn unit had the lowest cross-infection rate there was some disbelief. But true it was, and the protective clothes that we now see regularly on television during the present pandemic were one of the methods of reducing cross-infection which Paul and I had introduced to the unit when I arrived.

There were also connections with the paediatricians, which were not always friendly. Some paediatricians have an inborn belief that they must be in charge if the patient is a child, even when they know nothing about the medical or surgical problem. There were no issues with the consultants, Drs Raymond Brown and Cathy Noone, but their juniors would interfere with the drugs and in particular would prescribe unnecessary antibiotics. All of our staff would regularly point out that any severely burned person would automatically have a raised temperature as the natural way of fighting the injury, and this did not mean that it was caused by an infection. An unnecessary antibiotic could lead to resistance or the need for a later, more powerful antibiotic. Just after she was appointed Cathy joined us on a ward round to learn about burn care. A patient was presented, and it came out that the patient was a transexual fire-eater whose act had gone wrong. We pointed out that this was a normal burn patient – and I have not forgotten the look on Cathy's face.

Consultant Surgeon at Stoke Mandeville Hospital

When I started there were about four hundred admissions a year. Half of these were adults and half children, mostly under 5 years old. Very many of the families, particularly of the children, had major problems, and the children very rarely had married parents. The adults often had psychiatric, alcohol or drug problems and to a large extent had domestic injuries. Industrial injuries in Britain, even in major industrial areas, are low, unlike in many other countries, and even in America (*see* Chapter 9). Another problem that we always had to be aware of was non-accidental injuries. These were unfortunately not uncommon and needed very careful handling by all the staff. By the time I finished there, both because fewer people were having burn injuries, and because of the much shorter average stay, the unit was frequently half empty, and overflow patients from other wards often used the spare beds.

In summary, I enjoyed my time looking after burn patients and I feel that I contributed to their care and, through the research, to improvements. The nursing and additional inputs were marvellous and so was the contribution of most of the doctors. Being on call 24 hours a day, and often operating at weekends, was not a great hardship. If there was a problem very occasionally a senior nurse would gently phone me at home. I well remember one of these occasions when a new locum had been employed. I went into the hospital very rapidly, assessed the situation and suspended the doctor on the spot. On the Monday, expecting a problem, I was delighted when I was congratulated by the Management. It turned out that the doctor had been struck off by the General Medical Council and was using old references to find work. He then, need I say unsuccessfully, applied to be paid for the hours that he had worked!

After I retired, falling demand led to the unit being downgraded. It ceased to take major burn patients or young children with burns, and these were all sent to the three remaining large centres around us in Birmingham, Bristol and Chelmsford. I sometimes wonder why they did not try to do this when I was in post.

The next change in my workload came about through the National Spinal Injuries Unit. Stoke Mandeville was, and is, world famous as the first place in the world to have a specialist unit for the treatment of spinal injuries. Before the unit was created by Sir Ludwig Guttmann in 1944, patients with spinal injuries were left to become infected and to die, normally within weeks or a few months. Sir Ludwig was of Austrian Jewish background and had come out of Germany in 1939 to avoid the Nazi regime. He first worked in Oxford but was unable to find a post as a neurosurgeon – his actual specialty – and had started in Stoke Mandeville in 1941 with the dictum that patients with spinal injuries did not need to die, and through retraining and sport could become useful citizens. Apparently he had a German attitude to management and was very much a 'Dictator' with total care of the patient. He never took a holiday as that would have meant the loss of control. The unit that was to take spinal-injured military patients had twenty-six beds. It very rapidly had fifty patients. It was his naming of the unit in 1944, and raising money to build the Paralympic Stadium and the Paralympic Games, that cemented his reputation, and for which he was deservedly knighted. When I joined the hospital in 1985 there were three spinal consultants: Drs Isaac Nuseibeh, John Silver and Hans Frankel. I suggested that hand and arm surgery for the tetraplegics had a possible major use, and I went to Sweden to learn the techniques (*see* Chapter 9). Unfortunately I could not convince any of the consultants of the value of the surgery, but now, with new younger consultants in the Spinal Unit, some of the surgery is being done by my successor, Mr Tony Heywood.

However, what I could offer was the modern treatment of pressure sores with often extensive surgery, and a much more rapid healing of what was, and is, a common cause of sepsis and death in paralysed patients. Pressure sores are very common in spinal patients, and before Guttman were the commonest cause of death. Avoidance is achieved through good nursing and education of the patient, and I never saw a single pressure sore that had occurred in our hospital, for which congratulations indeed to the nursing care. A remarkable record. The pressure sores that I did see occurred either before the patient was admitted, or after discharge, when depression could occur and the patients relaxed their pressure relief movements. I also did whatever other surgery was needed for the patients on the unit, except for spinal surgery. An advantage with this work was that I used a spinal injuries session in the operating theatres and not one of my three allocated sessions.

About eighteen months after I had been appointed, Mr Brian Gardner was added as a fourth consultant. He had passed the exams of both the College of Physicians and the College of Surgeons. I was asked to assess and help his surgical skills. After a few months we all agreed that he would continue as the excellent physician that he was, and I would do the surgery. The marvellous story about Brian was that on his first Christmas day, when it was then normal for a consultant to carve the turkey for the patients and to serve the Christmas pudding, he poured brandy over the pudding and lit it. Unfortunately it was directly below a fire alarm sensor. The three fire engines and their crews that arrived very rapidly were thanked for their services, and then suitably fed and watered.

When I left in 2001 the NSIU held a special celebration for me, and I still have the elegant piece of glassware with which I was presented.

Within the hospital I operated with Mr Chris Smallwood, a general surgeon, on immediate breast reconstructions after excisions for cancer. When Dr Susan Burge was appointed as a new consultant dermatologist, she immediately suggested that we should do a joint clinic, and this continued for some years until she transferred to Oxford.

The final person who was absolutely essential was my secretary. Compared to other hospitals, at Stoke in my time we each had a secretary and mine was in a separate office from mine. One of my first jobs was to interview applicants for my new job. There were four formal applications and after their not very appealing interviews I was asked whether we could interview a fifth person who had just qualified as a medical secretary to give her interview experience. And in came Catherine. She interviewed brilliantly and she was appointed. She stayed with me for about four years until leaving to get married. She was always in the clinics and took shorthand. Her efficiency meant that I could see almost twice as many patients, and there were only small gaps between patients whilst a letter was dictated, or Catherine would say for standard cases, 'The usual letter I presume?'

When Catherine left to get married, I had three other secretaries for a few months or a year each. None of them did shorthand and the clinics suffered markedly. Finally Liz Neal, who had been in the Royal Air Force as a secretary and was very capable at shorthand, was appointed to the role and very excellent she was. Just after she started one morning she came into my office and said, 'Somebody is pulling my leg. There is someone on the phone saying that he is the Duke of Kent.' 'It will be,' I said. Luckily she had not put down the phone and I had a conversation with him. My standing rose immediately!

As well as my work in Stoke Mandeville, I also had NHS clinics in Reading, Northampton and later Buckingham, and operated in High Wycombe and Milton Keynes. Occasionally I had patients in RAF Halton (*see* Chapter 5) and in Oxford. Initially the clinics away from Stoke Mandeville took place on Friday afternoons.

I took over the rheumatoid hand surgery clinic at Reading from Bruce and worked there with Dr Francis Andrews. I had done very little of the sub-specialty before and therefore arranged to go to Wrightington Hospital in Lancashire to work with Professor John Stanley to learn the techniques involved in hand joint replacements. In Reading, Francis, having worked with Bruce for many years, was a little unsure about his new colleague, and the first patients he asked me to operate on were foot problems. Clearly I passed muster, and we worked together from 1985 until his retirement in 1991. Francis was an incredible person. A superb rheumatologist, he was also on the Council of the Royal College of Physicians, and was deeply loved by all his patients. He retired at the age of 60 to train as the equivalent of a priest in the Roman Catholic church. I do know that he was somewhat upset that he could not formally become a priest as he was married. He was perhaps even more upset that Church of England vicars who were transferring to the Catholic Church at that time were welcomed as priests, even though they were married. His retirement speech was fascinating. He was a severe diabetic and when he was diagnosed at school it was in the days when treatment was more hit and miss. He said that at the age of 12 he had heard the physician say to his parents that he would be very lucky to survive a year. 'Every year since has been a bonus,' was his comment. I came across his diabetes on occasions during clinics when he was going off slightly, and I would make him eat some biscuits and have a cup of sugared tea. I remember that the drive to Reading through the Chiltern woods on the first Friday of each month was very often the most beautiful and relaxing hour of the month.

The other clinic that I inherited was in the Northampton General Hospital on the second and third Fridays of each month. This started as a general plastic surgery clinic run concurrently with an SHO who was doing a minor operating list. There was an excellent secretary, Jayne Ponting, who ran the unit and was still in post when I retired.

Some years later I persuaded the local rheumatologist, Dr Tim Beer, that we should do a joint rheumatology hand clinic. There had been no previous rheumatoid hand surgery available, and by this time I had become totally convinced that there was an enormous amount of potential gain for the patients. Tim was less convinced at the beginning, but after some of my early patients had started talking in his clinics to other patients, there was unleashed a large potential workload as they all wanted operations. Now Tim was totally convinced, and over the next few years I worked through the backlog.

There were several benefits from rheumatoid hand surgery. Although the disease could not be cured, there were enormous gains both with the reduction in pain and also with an increase in function. One also got to know some patients well, partly because the surgery needed was often in several steps, and partly because the disease continued and would need further surgery in succeeding years. In comparison the normal plastic surgery patient one saw only once or perhaps twice (although there were exceptions, notably severely burned and melanoma cancer patients).

After a few months in post I was delighted to receive an invitation for my wife and me to dine with some of the Buckingham GPs. After an excellent dinner I discovered the reason for the invitation. In Buckingham there was a GP-run cottage hospital. They had somehow discovered that I had one Friday afternoon a month clear, and would I please do a clinic in their hospital. The effects of the alcohol made me accept the invitation, and the clinic continues to this day.

On occasions over the years I was asked to go to Milton Keynes Hospital to operate with the orthopaedic surgeon Mr John Lourie on serious leg injuries, and to High Wycombe Hospital to operate with Mr James Grogono on breast excisions for cancer with an immediate silicone implant. By chance James and I had known each other since we were both in short trousers as his father had been my GP in Essex, and also through sailing against each other at university matches.

The Oxford visits were to the Special Care Paediatric Unit, which looked after any baby with serious burns who was under a year old. If the patient needed surgery, I would operate there.

As well as the clinical work and the teaching (*see* Chapter 10), I collected a variety of extra posts over the years. I was also sent on two management courses at regional headquarters. Very surprisingly I was asked to consider being the Medical Director at Stoke, but I very quickly quashed that idea. I was also sent on two courses on 'Training the Trainers', from which I learned nothing new at all. The second one of these was to qualify as an instructor on future courses. There was another consultant surgeon on the latter whom I had not met before. We got on extremely well, and were somewhat unkind to a psychiatrist who was trying to control us. For some reason neither of us was asked to instruct on future courses!

There were other responsibilities too. Within the hospital in about 1990 an Audit Committee was founded of which I was made a member. Within the health service there were awards for exceptional service which were awarded on a national basis, at the various levels of A+, A, B and C. These were added to one's salary and were also pensionable. In my last three years I was the surgical representative on the that committee; at a regional level I was on the Plastic Surgery Advisory Committee, and for my last three years was chair of that committee. For surgical colleges I was made the surgical tutor in the hospital by the Royal College of Surgeons, and was also an elected member of the Council of the British Society for Surgery of the Hand. I was also appointed as an examiner for the Royal College of Surgeons of Glasgow and I held this position for twelve years (*see* Chapter 10).

My main work outside the hospital was with burn organisations. I was a member of the International Society for Burn Injuries and had been put on the Disaster Planning sub-committee. I should say that it never met in my time.

I was also a member of the British Burn Association (BBA) and organised their annual meeting at Stoke Mandeville in 1991. When I was on the committee a Burn Prevention Committee was formed, of which I was made chair. I had a very long-standing belief that the major way forward in burn care was education, and also, where necessary, changes to the law. Mr Douglas Jackson had done the original research in Birmingham which caused the selling of inflammable nightwear to be made illegal, and also for all electric fires to be guarded. The latter had an interesting history in that the original law required the guard to work for adult hands only, and it had to be modified to apply to small children as children's cases continued to occur. My involvement with this derived from my appointment as the BBA representative on the electrical section of the British Standards Institute. Some very interesting meetings followed, with clear differences of opinion between the manufacturers and those interested in safety. There were also problems with the European regulations and making all compatible. Whilst I was involved, one major change was the agreement to shorten the flex on kettles and other kitchen implements so that young children could not pull on a hanging down cable when they were climbing. This had often resulted in scalds from the hot water. This was the only occasion where the manufacturers instantly agreed, as it would save them money.

In the 1990s approximately 700 people a year in the UK died from burn injuries. Of these, about 400 of the fires were caused by cigarettes, and often with alcohol involved. Pipe tobacco goes out if the pipe is not being smoked, and it was known from the United States that this could also be the case in cigarettes, to which a chemical was added during manufacture to keep them alight when not being actively smoked. We therefore started a Fire Safe Cigarette campaign to try to have the law changed. Needless to say, the cigarette companies were violently against this as apparently 20–30 per cent of any cigarette burns away whilst not being actively smoked. They could see their profits decreasing and put up a variety of reasons why there should be no change, and this included the patently obviously fallacious argument that removing the chemical could make the cigarette more dangerous healthwise. They well knew that this would be almost impossible to prove without relevant research which would cost an enormous amount of money. We decided to launch a national TV and radio campaign, for which we obviously needed a well known figurehead. I first approached Esther Rantzen, with whom I had been in contact through 'That's Life' (*see* Chapter 10), and then Edwina Currie, who had done some fundraising for 'Restore', my research trust (*see* Chapter 3). Both said that they accepted that deaths could be reduced but they were total anti-smokers, and therefore could not support the campaign. Someone then suggested Ken Livingstone, the Labour MP, who instantly agreed. We held a TV briefing in the House of Commons, which was well received in the Press, but despite trying for another two years no final agreement with the tobacco companies could be reached. Looking back now I wonder where I found the time for all these extra commitments.

Although I had left my former career in engineering as the companies for whom I was working had tried to make me a manager, I had to accept that management was important. When I had been training, much of the management in the NHS was done by consultant physicians and surgeons who had an interest. This became less so as non-clinical managers were brought in. Many were of very poor quality as the pay was low by industry standards. Occasionally they were excellent. They included the hospital secretary when I joined and later Mr Ken Cunningham, our CEO. One of the problems with the managers was that they had no experience of patients. Ken, by contrast, had been a senior hospital laboratory technician in Glasgow and so knew about patients, and his excellence was partly due to this. In the ten years that we worked together one could always put up a case, and after discussion in 90 per cent of the cases he would agree with the change, or give good reasons why it was not possible. Ken was also a Formula 1 addict, and we would meet at Silverstone. And he kindly has written the Foreword for this book. The lay chair of the hospital was Mrs Gillian Miscampbell, whom I had met at my interview. She was an interesting person and a strong Tory supporter. I once asked her why she had not stood as a candidate for Parliament, and she told me that it would have made being a mother difficult. I am still in touch with both Gillian and Ken.

When Ken was promoted to manage a failing Trust his successor was, I thought, not in the same class. She once came into my office to demand that I operated on three long-waiting patients the next week. At that time there was a maximum waiting time for any operation, and if the management did not organise their surgery they would lose some or all of their bonus. There was also a somewhat contradictory, but very necessary, statement from Parliament that clinical need was to be prioritised. My response to the CEO was that I had three patients with cancer on my next list, and they were certainly going to have priority.

'What am I going to do about these long-waiters?'

'If you give me an extra operating list, I will be able to do them' was my answer. None was made available as it would have needed extra funding. I resigned from the NHS very soon after this and similar arguments.

* * *

One cannot write about Stoke Mandeville without some comments on the scandals which happened whilst I was there and within a few years afterwards.

The first that came to light after I had been in post for about two years was Dr Michael Salmon, a consultant paediatrician, who had amongst other things published an excellent and respected textbook. On considerable evidence he was prosecuted as a paedophile and sent to jail. Further evidence then came to light and his sentence was increased to a total of eighteen years.

Much has been said and written about Jimmy Savile. Whatever else he did, he did an enormous amount for the Spinal Unit at Stoke Mandeville and for spinal injuries worldwide. As a Bevin Boy during the Second World War he had suffered a spinal injury himself in the coal mines, from which he took some time to recover. The old spinal injury wards were collapsing in the 1970s, and he started to fundraise in 1972. He raised the amazing sum of £10 million, which enabled the new unit to be opened in 1983, and it is said that altogether for the unit and spinal research he raised as much as £40 million. Walking around the hospital I would often see a smiling Jimmy, and we would talk. A one-to-one conversation was interesting, but as soon as three or four people gathered, the act came on. When I set up the research trust I tried to get his help, but without success. On one Sunday my daughters had come with me to the hospital and were in my office whilst I did a ward round. I came across Jimmy and I said that my daughters wanted to meet him. 'Go and get them,' he said, which I did, and I took a photograph of Jimmy with one arm round each of them. At boarding school they kept this picture on their bedside table, until the scandal broke. At this point my financially inclined daughter asked me if she thought she could get some money out of the case. On another occasion he looked shattered. I asked him if he was OK, and he told me that he had finished his 99th marathon or half marathon the previous day and was feeling a little tired. And that was in a heavy smoker!

Hospitals are great places for rumours to spread easily. Whilst I was there, there were no rumours in the hospital about him misbehaving, and Ken and Gill have backed up this statement.

The third person accused of sexual abuse was my senior colleague, Bruce Bailey. I knew nothing about this until a journalist phoned me after I had retired and asked for a comment. I could only say that I had heard nothing about it and would be completely surprised if there was any truth in it. Certainly the case went no further.

Private Practice

My NHS contract allowed me one session a week for private practice. There were no financial costs to this until the private practice income became 10 per cent of the NHS salary, and then one lost that 10 per cent. There were also evenings and weekends available for private practice.

In my training very little concerning private practice was discussed. When I worked as a house surgeon in Cambridge, Bill Everett gave me a cheque every three months for clerking and looking after his patients on the ward, and in Bradford I was paid by Tom Barclay for operating on some of his patients. This also happened in Melbourne, where Bernie O'Brien would pay me for assisting or doing operations. But no one had given me any information on how to set up and run a private practice. Very soon after I started at Stoke Mandeville, BUPA (the largest medical insurance group in the UK) invited a group of new consultants to a day seminar on how to run a practice, and this was extremely useful.

There were three private hospitals around Aylesbury. Bruce Bailey worked in one, and Sanu Desai in another. I approached the third, the Chiltern Hospital in Wendover, and they were very pleased to see me, and even offered me the free use of a consulting room once a week for three months. I did no advertising but somehow referral letters started arriving. Cosmetic or aesthetic surgery was not my interest or skill, and I put these patients off. In fact in the whole of my career I have never done a facelift. The commonest groups of patients had skin tumours or carpal tunnel syndromes. Almost no patients with rheumatoid arthritis were covered privately, and with only two exceptions any privately insured burn patient was admitted to Stoke Mandeville, and the private insurance money went into the research funds.

In the early days I would do a clinic on Wednesday afternoons and then an operating list in the evening when I had sufficient patients. Whenever possible, Richard Bunsell was the anaesthetist. The referrals built up quite rapidly and it became clear that a part-time private secretary was necessary. I employed Carol Doyle, who looked after both the private patients and the medico-legal work (*see* Chapter 10). Within a few months I was also getting private referrals in Northampton, and I started a private clinic (but no operating) on some Friday evenings at the Three Shires Hospital.

One problem with my private practice was that my house was situated about 45 minutes' drive from the Chiltern Hospital to the south and also 45 minutes from the Three Shires Hospital to the north. Two options were possible. Some two years after moving in, I was rebuilding the farmhouse and barns that we had bought. It would be relatively easy to incorporate a consulting room, a waiting room, a secretary's office and a minor operating theatre into the changes. The second option was to use the Saxon Clinic, the private hospital in Milton Keynes, at least for operations. I chose both options. The Saxon Clinic had one great advantage in that it would organise a private operation at a guaranteed price, and then collect the fees both for myself and the anaesthetist. This was ideal for some patients, and particularly for breast enlargements. I used the hospital either on a Friday evening or on a Saturday once a month.

A further change that occurred was when we moved to The Old House in Whitchurch, and again into a barn I was able to add the same facilities, which included a minor operating theatre. My theatre sister at both of these houses was Jacky Benson, who was the senior plastic surgery theatre sister at Stoke Mandeville. I had two further changes of secretary too, first to Alyson Kirkham and finally to Penny Maier – and an excellent service all three provided.

The question arises: why do private practice at all? Firstly, there was a demand, as my operating and clinic times in the NHS hospitals were very limited. Secondly, the patients were often very interesting people, and this way one had a chance to get to know them far better. Several, indeed, I am still in contact with more than twenty years later. Names I cannot mention but some were household names. I remember two who were in the Chiltern for operations, and the nurses were queuing up to wheel them to theatre. Their names meant absolutely nothing to me but apparently they were both well known pop stars. I have added the stories of some of the patients to Chapter 11. And finally, it enhanced one's income very considerably. Was there a downside? It was a major commitment both for time, and also being on permanent call for any problems. On three evenings a week my wife and I would meet for dinner at about 10 o'clock.

There was also a social life involved, particularly with the Chiltern Hospital. This was an opportunity to meet colleagues from other hospitals. One of these was Alan Vass. We had met and got on well when I was a student at Oxford and he was the senior registrar in obstetrics and gynaecology. Medicine is a strange career. As one moves around the country with changing jobs it is very rare not to know someone in the new hospital. The Chiltern Hospital had a pitch and putt golf course and organised various competitions including an annual dog-show. One part of this was to find the owner who looked most like their dog, to the great amusement of the audience one year this was won by Geoffrey Channon, an orthopaedic surgeon at Amersham Hospital. Unfortunately, I do not have a photograph, but he bore a remarkable likeness to his Labrador.

* * *

What are now my thoughts about my sixteen years as a consultant at Stoke Mandeville? My interests within the speciality were agreed at the start, and as other interests developed there was only encouragement to continue with them. I also had encouragement with the research and with the military connections that built up. What I missed most was that I was not in a university setting and had no regular medical students to teach and to involve in the research. My overseas work made up for some of this, and I was extremely lucky to have been able to somehow fit it all in.

Aylesbury was in the country and my daily travel into the hospital, and more especially my travel to my other NHS clinics and to the private hospitals was restful and enjoyable. By the time I retired Aylesbury had grown enormously, and I was not too sad to leave our lovely fifteenth-century house which had once stood on a quiet road, but that was no longer the case. My wife Vivian had found a marvellous general practice which had thrived enormously through her work.

I had been very lucky indeed to have been appointed to the post at Stoke Mandeville.

Chapter 3

Research

Before I started medicine I had had a background of research during my engineering life. I had done three years of research at Cambridge University, was a lecturer in engineering at the University of Surrey for three years, and also worked in industrial research for the Shell Research Company, for the Coke Research Association and for ICI.

During my time as a medical student the importance of research in medicine was constantly discussed at Oxford. During the six years whilst I was qualifying and registering as a doctor I was not involved in any research. When I started my SHO post in the Accident Service in Oxford I planned a research project. It was approved by Mr John Cockin, the consultant orthopaedic surgeon in charge of the accident service, and I started to do the work with Peter Teddy, who had been a medical student in my year and had already been involved in research and had a PhD in neurophysiology. We had started working in the accident service one month apart. The project was to determine whether giving antibiotics to patients with hand injuries reduced the incidence of infection. The result showed no evidence of a reduction in hand laceration infection after using antibiotics, which were both painful and could lead to penicillin resistance. Following our paper, the use of penicillin in hand injuries has now mostly stopped. What did matter was keeping the bandages dry.

I had been involved in research at the Birmingham Accident Hospital during my training which led to what is now the universal use of superglue both to fix skin grafts and to close wounds.

Whilst in Newcastle I became very involved in the treatment of hypospadias, a common congenital abnormality of boys, and I devised two new operations and also collected information about its prevalence. The work done at Oxford showed that the use of antibiotics in hand lacerations had no useful gain. In Newcastle I set up a further trial using povidone iodine as a prophylactic antiseptic treatment instead of penicillin in what was basically the same trial, and this did show an advantage in reducing postoperative wound infection.

Before leaving an extremely busy job in Newcastle, I did a two month locum at East Grinstead, where I met some of the consultants involved and also members of the Guinea Pig Club. The club had been set up and named by severely burned airmen who in the Second World War had been operated on by Sir Archibald McIndoe. As well as his brilliant surgery, he was very involved in getting the badly scarred patients accepted into as normal a life as possible. There are several books about the club which are well worth reading. Whilst I was there I had the time to write two papers on hypospadias repair as it was a less busy job.

During my appointment in Yorkshire both the consultants in Bradford, Mr Barclay and Mr Crockford, were extremely keen and supportive of trainee surgeons doing research and publishing the results. Mr Barclay had introduced tissue expansion to this country as a method of stretching skin, and also a new method of using extended skin flaps for the same purpose. With help from three of the trainees, the results and the complications were measured and published. During this time I also wrote papers on melanomas and other skin tumours, on the surgery of burns and on hand injuries. In 1985 the Bradford Football Club fire occurred, and my experience of this was published as a paper and a booklet. In total from my four years in Yorkshire I published ten papers and a book chapter.

As discussed in Chapter 1, in July 1981 I started a year's fellowship in Melbourne, Australia. The primary purpose was to train to be able to do microsurgery, but in addition I had the opportunity to be involved in the unit's research. I became involved in studying the effects and the potential value of using vasodilating drugs on the outcomes. I was also involved in their work on lymphoedema, and its possible correction by microsurgery. The blood flow studies were going very well until the apparatus broke down and could not be repaired or replaced before my year finished. The early results had been exciting, and the final work would have been published as a thesis for a higher degree. The results are now used in clinical practice, but were never formally published. One paper was published on the lymphoedema studies and another on the treatment of microvascular grafts. And here I will admit that I wrote more papers on the ornithology of Australia than on the medical research!

When I started at Stoke Mandeville in 1985, a session each week for research and teaching had been built into my contract. I decided that the most useful way of using this was to produce small research projects for the junior trainee surgeons who were working in the unit, which they could do in addition to their normal training programme. This worked

Research

very well for fifteen years, during which time the unit produced eighteen scientific papers in a variety of surgical journals. The majority of this work was based on clinical problems from admissions to the unit.

Over the next few years it became evident to me, particularly in the Burn Unit, that there were also sufficient projects available for one or more full-time research fellows. A one-year Fellowship for a higher surgical degree was then of great benefit to trainee surgeons wishing to advance through the ranks to become a consultant, and also it opened up the possibility of doing important research with a clinical use. To employ research Fellows one needed firstly a project, then sufficient money to pay them, and also to pay for their laboratory space and equipment. I therefore looked at the possibilities of setting up a research trust. I decided to discuss the possibility of creating an independent research trust with the chair of the hospital board, Mrs Gillian Miscampbell. Her view was that this would be a sensible way forward. The next thing to do was to create a legally sound trust and to have it approved by the Charity Commissioners. After doing some research, it was clear that the first thing I had to do was find some trustees and a chair from amongst them. I then needed a patron and vice-patrons. I started with the trustees, and I was extremely lucky that all of the people that I approached agreed to take on the responsibility. They were Mrs Miscampbell, Mr Bruce Bailey, Sir Desmond Fennell, a High Court judge, the Lady Alexander of Weedon, Gavin Campbell, who was the number two presenter for the television series 'That's Life' and with whom I had done some television work, and finally Professor Sir Ronald Mason. Ronald had been the Chief Scientific Adviser to the Ministry of Defence and was a Fellow of the Royal Society. He had recently retired and agreed to chair the trustees. All of them were either colleagues from within the hospital or themselves (or a family member) had been one of our patients. Because of a family member who had been a patient, the Earl of Inchcape, who was a local landowner, agreed to be our Patron. I then approached various people to be vice-patrons and everybody except one agreed to take on the role. The only person who did not was Richard Branson, who very reasonably said that he was already supporting several charities and thought it inappropriate to take on another. The vice-patrons included four members of the House of Lords, Sir Edward Tomkins, a former British ambassador in France, and my own Professor of Medicine, Sir Richard Doll. He wrote me a very nice letter saying that of course he would support any of his old students who wished to be involved in research. Richard Doll had proved the causation of lung cancer by smoking and although he was world famous, he was never given the Nobel prize that he so richly deserved. The other vice-patrons were another colleague, Sanu Desai, Sir Evelyn de Rothschild and Sir Andrew Hugh-Smith. It was a very impressive list of well-known names both nationally and locally. It was not until many years later, when I was assessing applications for another charity for funding, that I realised how lucky I had been by chance. When an application came into the other charity, the first thing that I and the other assessors would do was to look at the list of Patron, vice-patrons and trustees on the letterhead. Then we looked at what previous research had been done and published, and the last thing that we did was to look at the project for which funding was being requested.

The next thing was to choose a name for our trust which had to say as clearly as possible to donors what the trust was doing. The decision was to call it the Stoke Mandeville Burns and Reconstructive Surgery Research Trust (later to be renamed 'Restore – Burn and Wound Research' when it became of national importance). We all agreed that the original was somewhat long winded, but could not think of anything shorter that was more appropriate. Horwood & James, a firm of solicitors in Aylesbury, very kindly offered to carry out the legal necessities for the creation of the trust and its registration with the Charity Commissioners at no charge. They have continued to provide legal services on the rare occasions that we have needed them since, again for no charge, and for which my thanks.

My senior colleague Mr Bruce Bailey had over the years been donated sums for research totalling approximately £120,000 by grateful patients and this was held in the NHS accounts of the hospital. There was considerable doubt as to whether this could be moved from the NHS to the trust account, but with the aid of Mrs Miscampbell it happened. The trustees met to discuss possible future fundraising, and also to agree that we should advertise for our first research Fellow.

The policy for raising money was decided. As well as local fundraising events, there would be applications to trusts and other charities that might have money available. A decision was made not to employ fundraisers, based on the experience of two other medical research charities where very rapidly the cost of raising the money became more than the money successfully raised. We very soon discovered that chance was a major factor. We held a tea party at the abbey in Aston Abbotts which raised some £400. The next day I had a telephone call from one of the people who was at that tea party saying that he had been impressed with the work we were doing, and his company would offer us £10,000. On another occasion I and my wife were at a dinner with friends in a small restaurant when a man sitting at the next table, who had obviously been listening to our conversation, invited himself and his wife to join us for coffee. Following the conversation, a trust of which he was the major donor subscribed £25,000 a year for ten years to fund a research Fellow. We also had a major anonymous donor on several occasions in those early years. The events were always useful in keeping our work in the news locally, but were not always financially useful. With the backing of Lord Alexander, the President of the MCC, we had for instance two cricket matches where a team of surgeons played the Old England Test Team XI. They certainly attracted press attention, but only raised a few hundred pounds each time. We also found that we required laboratory space and special tests on an increasing basis as the research became more specialised. Some of the work was at University College Hospital, London and at Cambridge University, but by far the greatest laboratory use was in the medical school in Oxford. This laboratory use was expensive, and almost doubled the amount of money needed for each Fellow when added to their salary. The supervision of the research was originally under my direction, but as it became more specialised help was given by Professor McGrouther at University College Hospital, London and by Professor Harris in Oxford. They both spent many hours supervising the Fellows and made no charges to the Trust.

Two years later a patient of mine insisted on joining us to help our research. Peter Chapman had been a champion motor-cycle racer, having won the Isle of Man TT sidecar championship many years earlier. He brought enormous enthusiasm and some marvellous connections to the trustees. He organised fundraising events for us at Silverstone during several Formula 1 Grand Prix, which were both lucrative and great fun. Nigel Mansell, the World Champion, presented me with a large cheque (not his own money!). Peter also recruited John Surtees to be a vice-patron. John was the only person to be world champion at both motor-cycle road racing and Formula 1 car racing, and whenever he was doing a book signing we were always very grateful when the proceeds came to us, until his death in 2017.

The next person to join us, and I still do not know why, was Mrs Amanda Nicholson, who was High Sheriff of Buckinghamshire at the time. She was very welcome indeed and had excellent connections around the county, and her husband John organised various events for us.

Our first patron, the 3rd Earl of Inchcape, died in 1994 and we needed to find a replacement. I had met HRH the Duke of Kent on several occasions when skiing and when we were both staying with the vice-patron Sir Edward Tomkins and Lady Tomkins in their chalet in Meribel. Having told the Duke about the research that we were doing, I asked him if he would become our patron. To my delight and surprise, he agreed and said that he would be our patron for five years. Nearly thirty years later he is still our patron (see Plate 3.1). We arranged that he would come to Stoke Mandeville Hospital to meet some of our patients and the Burn Unit staff, and then to my house to meet and thank some of our vice-patrons, trustees and donors. He told me afterwards that he had been very worried how he would react to seeing badly burned people, but had found it interesting. I never told him that the patients whom he met on his first visit were carefully selected by me to be some of the less seriously burned or injured. What becomes normal to doctors and nurses over some years is often shocking to somebody who is not used to seeing severe deformity or scarring, even when they have been in the Army. The Duke's visits to Stoke Mandeville became an almost annual event and were very much appreciated by patients and staff. When he came to our house for the evening event, I was surprised that he asked for a room on his own for thirty minutes; I later discovered that in this time he read and learned the five-line summaries of all of the people that he was about to meet. Most members of the royal family work extremely hard. Many years later I asked him, 'When do you retire?' To which he answered, 'An interesting question – nobody has ever asked me that before.' He is still working.

Over the years the Duke also attended meetings at the Royal Society and the Royal Society of Medicine, both in London, where our research was being presented.

The trustees have changed too, after the deaths of several, including Sir Desmond Fennell, Mr Peter Chapman and Mr Bruce Bailey. James Naylor joined us around the same time, and with Ron Mason, now recently deceased, has been our longest-serving trustee. Mike Constant, a local friend in Buckinghamshire, took over the chair from Ron Mason and he was followed by Lord Calum Graham and now by Mike Tyler. Mike was our second Fellow – so it has come full circle.

The vice-patrons have also changed with the deaths of several, including Sir Richard Doll, Lord Carrington, Sir Edward Tomkins, John Surtees, Lord Kearton and Lord Hartwell. My very sincere thanks to all those who have helped over the thirty years.

Research

Although the clinical work on the patients was still at Stoke Mandeville Hospital, the laboratory work was being carried out in Cambridge, in Oxford and at University College in London. The fundraising also became more national. A decision was made to change the name of the trust. With the help of Mrs Nicholson, a company was recruited to do this and eventually it was agreed that we would become 'Restore – Burn and Wound Research'. I still think that my suggestion of 'SABRE – Scar And Burn Research' was better. And it would have been much cheaper!

A decision had been made that laboratory animals would not be used. The research did become more laboratory based using modern scientific apparatus to analyse human specimens. Professor Gus McGrouther, at the time the only Professor of Plastic Surgery in the United Kingdom, and an old friend and colleague of mine, became very much involved and much of the subsequent success of the research for the next fifteen years can be attributed to him.

The research Fellows (later to be called The Duke of Kent Fellows) have always been appointed at a competitive interview after shortlisting. This has normally been for a one-year appointment, but Jonathan Pleat did three years for his D Phil degree. When the finances or the awards of scholarships allowed, we often had more than one Fellow at any time.

Our first Fellow, Ali Juma, was appointed to the post to work on the return of sensation following partial or full thickness grafting of burned skin. The next nine Fellows worked on the topic of burn depth and its modification, with some success. The old method of diagnosing the depth of a burn was in degrees: 1st degree was sunburn or similar, 2nd degree was a superficial burn, or part way through the skin, and 3rd degree was a full thickness burn. More severe 4th, 5th and 6th degree burns – the latter to bone – had been described, but the terms were no longer used. Mr Douglas Jackson, the world burn expert from the Birmingham Accident Hospital, had noticed, however, that some superficial burns healed with no scarring in ten days, while some took three or four weeks to heal and scarred, often severely. He termed these superficial partial thickness and deep partial thickness burns. They could normally be separated by examination, but the actual difference in the damage or the body's response to the damage had not been discovered. Clearly if there was a definite difference and the deep partial burn could be made into a superficial burn, then an operation would not be necessary and no scarring would result. Mike Tyler and Andy Watts discovered that the difference occurred when a specific depth through the skin had been damaged, and this was a remarkably consistent figure of 23 per cent, irrespective of the original thickness of the skin, which varies enormously between, for instance, the back and an eyelid. We then tried methods of modifying this depth. Paul Banwell started by applying a vacuum to the surface. This was being developed for aiding the healing of skin ulcers. Although very effective for ulcers, it made no difference to the burn healing. Further work was done by Titus Adams on the effect of suction. James Murphy used a drug which inhibited a chemical found in burned skin. This worked well, but only in the short term. Professor McGrouther then developed a method of putting a small incision of varying but known depth in normal skin and Chris Dunkin used this for further studies on the effect of depth on the healing of normal skin. From samples taken from this, Jonathan Pleat used a completely different technique to elucidate the different proteins that were released by injuries at different depths, and he has also continued supervising later Fellows. At the end of this research much more is known about the burning and the healing process, but no long-term solution has yet been found to reduce the scarring. Research is still continuing.

Another Fellow, Liz Hormbrey, used a similar technique to analyse the effect of healing following breast reconstruction.

Early cooling of a burn injury is known to be effective in reducing the depth of a burn and is more effective than would be expected on a temperature basis alone. Work is still continuing, and a study of the reasons for this effect is progressing well.

Research has been an important and very interesting part of my life. As with all research, much of it will contribute nothing to clinical work in the future, but some of my published papers have been useful, and are quoted in the literature and have become standard practice. The work has also been the cause of many of my overseas invitations to present the work. All proceeds from this book will be given to the Trust.

Chapter 4

Early Military Involvement

In the introduction I mentioned that my father had joined the Royal Air Force Volunteer Reserve at the beginning of the Second World War as an administrative Pilot Officer. What his duties were I can only imagine, but no doubt they were similar to those of all admin officers now – but with pen and ink and no computer. He was first stationed at RAF Lossiemouth and was for a time at RAF Grange-over-Sands, and finished up as the adjutant at RAF Benson with the rank of squadron leader. No real memories remain except for the various hospitals that I attended. It would be marvellous to say that I remembered planes taking off on bombing raids and then some returning – but my only memories of these events was from the films that I saw later.

Towards the last days of the war, by which time my parents had in effect parted, I remember hearing a V1 Doodlebug, and then its engine turning off. But there is no memory of the subsequent crash and explosion, which could have been some miles away. I also remember seeing the devastation caused by a V2 rocket which landed close to my Aunt Dot's house in Chadwell Heath in Essex, and also watching floodlights picking up German bombers over London. My next memory is of VJ day, when we celebrated in the park at Romford with Aunt Dot and Uncle Len Smoothy. He had recently been discharged from the Royal Naval Reserve in which he had served as an able seaman throughout the war.

When I went to Bancroft's School my actual involvement with the military commenced. At school it was expected that one joined either the CCF (the Combined Cadet Force) or the school sea scouts, and the majority of my year did one or the other, and only a few, mainly for medical reasons, did neither. I was already involved with the scouts at my church. I therefore joined the CCF. At our school the CCF involved only the Army and the Royal Air Force. Virtually all of the masters had either served during the war or had done national service. Several of them therefore were involved with the CCF. I am now not certain as to the logistics, but in memory in overall control was Sergeant Major West. Certainly he was the person who dished out the uniforms and was very much in control of teaching us to march and shoot and all of the other parts of the military life. He had been a sergeant major in the Parachute Brigade during the war and had done more than eighty jumps. I have never discovered whether he was actually a master at Bancroft's and funded by the school, or whether the army paid him. Certainly the Army part of the CCF wore the Parachute Brigade badge on our arm.

For the first year one was in the Army cadets. Friday afternoon was the time for the cadets or the scouts, and for the Army cadets this involved lectures and practical work, marching, arms and shooting on the .22 indoor range in the school grounds. Drill was learning to stand to attention, at ease and easy, and to march both slow and at normal speed, and to carry out the various manoeuvres involved, and I found it really quite interesting. I do remember Tim Pullen in my year having considerable problems. For some reason he insisted on the arm and foot on the same side moving together, rather than opposite to each other. This caused some consternation with Sergeant Major West, and considerable amusement to the rest of us. During his national service Tim became a pilot in the Royal Air Force, so his coordination could not have been as bad as we had thought in our first year. The other episode that we devised to upset the sergeant major and the officers was to practise privately American methods of drill. And when we tried these out on the parade ground it certainly did upset Sergeant Major West, but he took it well.

About once a month there was a field day (or more accurately, an afternoon rather than a whole day). Instead of our formal uniform we were allocated army field uniform, which we wore while we practised crawling, attacking and hiding in Epping Forest, which surrounded the school. Field days in good weather were great fun, and the only disadvantage was that we wore the same army boots. For the usual Friday afternoon parade these had, of course, to be immaculate, but at the end of a field day, particularly in the winter, they looked extremely scruffy indeed. They therefore had to be cleaned and polished for the next Friday afternoon parade. Cleaning and polishing boots takes a long time and a lot of effort to get a good result. I worked out, however, that if one used sandpaper followed by Valspar black lacquer, and then, when that dried, a coat or two of boot polish the result was extremely good. In fact it was so good that on the annual inspection an inspecting general took a look at my boots and said, 'Did you do those yourself?' I answered 'Yes sir' and he said, 'Well done.' At least my experimental method worked well and saved me many hours of polishing.

During the summer vacation at the end of my first year we all went off to camp. In that first year it was at Grimes Graves, which was a very large army camp in the scrublands of Norfolk. The reason why it was so large was that this was of course the time of National Service, and the camp was a major training area for new recruits. As well as the Bancroft's contingent, there were CCF contingents from several other schools, and immediately there developed a sense of rivalry between them and us. This was, of course, encouraged, and was manifest on the sports fields, on parade and on the shooting range. At school we had only fired .22 rifles. At Grimes Graves we moved onto a full-size outdoor range shooting Lee Enfield .303 rifles. Certainly every round fired gave a considerable thump into the shoulder at our tender age of 11 or 12. I was very successful as a marksman, although I very soon developed my own method of shooting. At this time I did not wear glasses but had noticed that my right eye was less focused than the left. I therefore shot left-handed, which with a .303 rifle was very difficult as the bolt to load the next round was designed for right-handed people. The method was tolerated by the NCO running the range as clearly it was effective for me. As well as formal shooting with real bullets, we also used blanks in the rifles when we were doing exercises in the low scrub and woodland. I remember the area was infested with rabbits and I worked out that putting a pencil up the spout of the rifle gave one a good chance of hitting a rabbit using only the blank as a propellant. I will say that I have never shot an animal since.

There was considerable rivalry between the various schools, which obviously caused some problems for the masters trying to control us. The riot act was read on several occasions. One night all was quiet. However, when the car containing three or four masters which had been parked outside our barrack rooms to ensure our good behaviour came to drive away, they discovered that somehow all four tyres had gone flat. I think it is fair to say that they were not amused, and we never did discover which school had done the deed – but, of course, it was not us.

That first year was useful in that one learnt a sense of discipline and developed a considerable toughness in outdoor conditions in the forest in the cold and bad weather, and the mud.

The other introduction that I had that year was playing the flute in the Corps of Drums. Volunteers were requested to learn the bugle, the drums or various woodwind instruments, of which only the B-flat and F flutes and the piccolos were within our school corps. The equipment, music and tuition were all provided, and it really was a no-brainer to join up. Within a few months we were happily marching up and down and leading the rest of the cadets. Given a flute now, I think I could still play the national anthem and 'Ash Grove', which seemed to be the most popular piece of music that we all learned at the beginning. My Aunt Dot was once visiting us and picked up my flute and tried to play it. Although a lot of air came out of her lips, no noise came out of the flute, and she was blowing so hard that she almost fainted. At least she did not go into tetany.

At the end of that first year we had to make a decision: to stay in the Army cadets or to join the Royal Air Force section. There was no naval section, as those who were interested in the sea had already joined the school sea scouts. In my mind there was no doubt that I would much prefer the Royal Air Force to the Army. And so I changed my khaki uniform for the Royal Air Force blue uniform. The training was considerably different. More time was spent in lectures, learning the basics of navigation, aircraft recognition and basic engine mechanics. The school also had a very crude elastic-powered glider situated at the playing grounds in West Grove, South Woodford. The glider was powered by two rubber bungees and a line of cadets would pull on each one to full extension; at this point the cadet acting as pilot pulled the release mechanism and the glider, if one was very lucky, flew for about 30 or 40 yards. Parade ground exercises continued, as did shooting, and we sat examinations in what we had been taught in the lectures.

But what we were all eagerly looking forward to was getting up into the air in an Air Force plane. In our first two years this happened only at the annual camps – a whole week spent on an RAF station. I remember camps at RAF Bassingbourn, RAF Manston and two stations in Lincolnshire. The planes commonly used for giving cadets flying experience were the Anson, the Oxford, the Chipmunk and the Proctor. And if we were very lucky, and particularly in the latter, we were given control of the plane to keep it flying level and make simple turns, but no acrobatics were allowed as the aircraft were not suitable. As well as the actual flying, all of the camps had flight training modules and we were all able to try out and hone our skills on these.

And then, in our third year, life changed. The inspecting officer that year was Group Captain Al Deere, a very famous New Zealand Battle of Britain Spitfire pilot, At that time he was commanding RAF North Weald, which was our local airfield, 12 miles north of school. He was

Early Military Involvement

obviously impressed by our turnout because at the end of the inspection he said that at any time if any of us wished to cycle up to North Weald we would be welcome, and he promised us a flight in some plane or other. In fact this was extremely unfair on the boarding members of the cadets, as school regulations prevented them from cycling. Nevertheless I, though surprisingly few of my fellow cadets, went up there on a regular basis.

My first visit was certainly interesting. I arrived at the guardhouse in my cadet uniform and said that Group Captain Deere had invited me or any RAF cadet from Bancroft's School to visit at any time. There was a certain degree of consternation but eventually the duty officer appeared. I explained what I was doing there and he, with no objection, took me into the officers' mess and introduced me to some of the pilots there. North Weald at that time was an interesting airfield. The resident 111 Squadron was then flying Meteors and provided the Royal Air Force aerobatic team. They were known as the Black Arrows and were the forerunners of the Red Arrows. The other two squadrons based there were 601County of London Squadron RAF and 604 County of Middlesex Squadron RAF. In the 1950s these were both very active at weekends with experienced and qualified pilots going back to North Weald to keep up their flying skills. These pilots were obviously older than the 111 Squadron pilots and were often much easier to talk to. Both squadrons were also flying Meteor 8s, the standard fighter in those days, along with the Vampire. There were also training planes based there and these included an Anson, an Oxford and a Meteor 7 twin-seater, as well as one Vampire twin-seater. Over the next few months I had flights in all of these except the Vampire, which unfortunately went unserviceable on the two occasions when I was about to fly in it. The outstanding flight was in the Meteor 7 doing aerobatics with 111 Squadron. After being thrown all over the sky by my pilot, who was the second in command of the squadron, he broke away from the formation and handed the controls to me. I had flown, looped and rolled a jet trainer, but having lined it up to land he had the sense to take over and landed it himself. I believe there are no longer any Meteor 7s in existence in England, but some years ago, whilst visiting Woomera in Australia, I saw one in the aircraft museum there and nostalgia came back with some force.

As well as the annual camps and my extra visits to North Weald, there was also the possibility of extra camps during the school vacations. I went to two of these in Royal Naval Air Stations. The first was HMS Daedalus at Lee-on-the-Solent in Hampshire. Clearly this was not all about flying, and we had an introduction to torpedoes, air sea rescue (including a trip into the Solent on a high-speed air sea rescue boat), as well as a flight in a De Havilland 89B Dominie biplane. Luckily I managed to be allocated the co-pilot's seat and therefore took over for part of the flight. In the back one of the other cadets was panicking on what was his first flight, and unfortunately several of the others were baiting him. Every time they saw a bonfire on the ground they told him that it was the other plane that had just crashed. He was not a happy lad. We were also due to have a helicopter flight but the chopper became unserviceable, and it was many years before I had my first helicopter flight. Another memory of that week was of a PT instructor, who, like many PT instructors, was not the kindest of men. Early one morning he had all the cadets on the parade ground and we were told to follow what he was doing. He held his arms parallel to the ground, either in front or to his sides and was rotating them in small circles, flexing the wrists or doing a series of other movements without at any time lowering his arms. It was extremely tiring, and one by one the cadets gave up and were subjected to his unfriendly comments. However, the three of us from Bancroft's were all extremely fit and only one of us gave up before the instructor himself gave up. The two of us remaining smiled, but unfortunately did not have the nerve to make a suitable comment. My other memory there was that the leading seaman who was overseeing the instruction offered us the examination paper that we would have to sit at the end of the week. We gave him in exchange a couple of drinks in the NCOs' mess. Perhaps not surprisingly we all passed with flying colours.

The second extra camp was at HMS *Blackcap*, the Royal Naval Air Station at Stretton in Lancashire. It was similar to the Lee-on-the-Solent camp but away from the sea. My main memory is of seeing a row of Seafires, the naval equivalent of the Spitfire. I remember asking one of the NCOs what they were going to do with the Seafires, and he said they were scrapping them, and that if we wanted to help ourselves we could go and take any part we liked. Unfortunately I only had a pocket knife with me but I am still the proud possessor of the firing button of a Seafire. How I wish that I had had more tools and time then, and even more that I had had the money to buy one of them as scrap. It would now be worth many hundreds of thousands of pounds. The other remarkable thing about this week was meeting a cadet from Oundle School named Barry Hook. We met again at Sea View Yacht Club in 1962, and remained firm friends until his death in 2018.

Early Military Involvement

The final part of my first admission to the Royal Air Force was when I attempted to gain a flying scholarship. If successful, I would have learned to fly and would automatically have become a pilot during my National Service. I would in fact very happily have had to sign on for the three years instead of the normal two years of National Service. I therefore filled out the relevant forms, received the backing of the school cadet force and went for selection to RAF Hornchurch. This was a three-day selection course which involved various tests of one's physical, mental and leadership abilities and a very full medical. In the afternoon of the third day I had a meeting with a wing commander who gave me the very good news that I had done exceptionally well in the ability tests, passing in the top 1 per cent of recruits, and then the very bad news that unfortunately I had failed the medical on my eyesight. I was short-sighted in my right eye and astigmatic in my left. Aircrew required perfect eyesight and glasses were not allowed. In those day corneal correction by lasers had not been invented, and even today it is only allowed for aircrew who have been fully trained and whose eyesight has then become less than perfect. The other potential problem for me was that having done well in the mental abilities tests, I might have been made a navigator and not a pilot. This happened to my son-in-law's father, who reached the grand rank of air commodore but is still slightly upset that he did not become an air marshal, which would have been far more likely had he been a pilot as they were, and are, preferentially promoted. And like him, I would have been less happy as a navigator than as a pilot.

Having failed to get the flying scholarship and a guaranteed slot in the Royal Air Force, I then had to decide what to do about my upcoming National Service. Did I go straight from school to do it, or did I go to university first? I had been put off by the experience of my cousin Alan, who went into the Royal Signals and to Catterick for initial training. Having volunteered to go anywhere around the world, he spent the whole of his two years at Catterick doing virtually nothing. It was an almost complete waste of two years. I also knew that with an engineering degree I would automatically be selected for officer training, which was by no means guaranteed entering directly from school. I therefore asked for deferment and this was granted. I still have the card confirming that I had been deferred. An interesting story was told to me by a friend, David Secker Walker. Prior to his first day on parade, he had been advised that when the sergeant major ordered anyone who played rugby at school to step forward, he should do so. It turned out, amazingly, that this was an automatic selection method for officer training, for which he was duly selected. The even more interesting fact was that David had been at Westminster School and played soccer, not rugby. But he got away with it and became an officer.

Off to university I went, with many happy memories of my time as a cadet in the services but with no commitment to join the officer training school at university. I did go to the university officers' mess on a couple of occasions, and as with all first-time attenders finished up with a pint of beer being poured down my trouser leg while I was doing a handstand. They were a pleasant group but I decided not to join. Do I regret this now? I really don't know. Having become involved with the military later in my career, I think that perhaps I would have enjoyed a military career. However, the great problem of being in the military is that to a very large extent one's choice as to the path that career will take may be outside the wishes or experience of the person.

At least four of the lads who were in my year at school joined the Royal Air Force as aircrew. The closest of my school friends, Roger Whitely, became a helicopter pilot and was unfortunately killed on duty. Another close friend, Gordon Heath, became a navigator on Vulcan bombers and remained in the Royal Air Force for the whole of his working life. Whilst at university I visited him on at least two occasions on the airfields where he was based. And again, some sadness about what I had not been able to do because of my eyesight became apparent.

Chapter 5

Military Involvement as a Surgeon

Although I had some military connections as a boy and as a young man, in my adult life I had no other military connections for many years until I was a surgical registrar at the Birmingham Accident Hospital. The senior surgeon on the trauma side was Mr Peter London, who had been a surgeon in the army during the war. He had a regular supply of military personnel coming to the hospital for instruction in the management of accidents. The ones I remember well were from the Special Air Service (SAS), and it was always interesting to congratulate them on their suntans though for some reason they would never tell us where they had acquired them. In my third year at Birmingham I made enquiries about becoming a part-time military surgeon, although I do not now remember why. I had an interview with the local commandant of the Royal Naval Reserve, and he said there was certainly a vacancy in the RNVR for somebody with my background and I could be attached to the Royal Marines (who do not have their own medical staff). This would have meant doing the green beret course and also basic training at Dartmouth. I filled out the various forms, but then was promoted to Newcastle and my application went no further.

There were then many years when I had no military involvement until I became the Director of the Oxford Regional Burn Unit at Stoke Mandeville Hospital. The main transport base for the Royal Air Force was at RAF Brize Norton, just to the west of Oxford, and the transport base for the United States Air Force was at RAF Upper Heyford, just to the north-east of Oxford. The proximity of both of these stations to the hospitals at Oxford and at Stoke Mandeville meant that when the First Gulf War began in August 1990 we were very involved in the planning and preparations to take the trauma cases to Oxford and the burns and spinal injury cases to Stoke Mandeville. The plan for Stoke Mandeville was that we should take the first hundred major burn patients. Using my experience from the Bradford Football Stadium fire and from the Athens petroleum refinery fire, and with the assistance of my colleagues and the administration, I worked out how this was to be done. I called on various burn consultant surgeons around the country, but in particular knew that the real problem of dealing with unexpectedly large numbers of patients with serious burns was the shortage of specialised nursing. I therefore reached the agreement that some recently retired nurses would come back to work, and that other nurses from burn units in the south of England would be transferred to Stoke Mandeville. Another problem that I foresaw was that some patients might have serious orthopaedic injuries as well as burn injuries. These would be assessed on admission as to which injuries were the more severe, and the patient then admitted to the appropriate hospital. Straightaway it was realised by Oxford that there was some lack of knowledge of dealing with serious burns. I was therefore asked to go to Oxford to give a series of lectures on the management of burns. It was somewhat strange to be the lecturer rather than a student in the 300-seat lecture theatre, and lecturing to many of the consultants who had taught me some fifteen years previously.

During this same time I had a request from the United States Air Force to assess the burn care provision in two of their three emergency hospitals based in Britain. These were at RAF Upper Heyford and RAF Little Rissington. Both had been set up at very short notice, and were close to the main transport link for the US Air Force. Because of the distance involved in evacuating casualties from Saudi Arabia or the Gulf states back to the United States, these two emergency hospitals were to be a staging post. My first visit was to RAF Upper Heyford, where I met Colonel Miller, the medical commander there. He was a delightful, tall, black consultant gynaecologist. They had set up a burn unit, which amazingly included a saline bath – a technique that had been developed during the Second World War but had been superseded as a method in burn care some twenty years later. During my visit, in conversation with Colonel Miller and his colleagues, it became apparent that there were no doctors or nurses with any experience of burn care to care for burn patients. It also became apparent that there was a considerable rivalry with RAF Little Rissington as to which hospital would look after such patients. Very clearly neither hospital wanted the responsibility. I then gave some formal lectures and a considerable amount of informal teaching before leaving. Just before I left, Colonel Miller presented me with the squadron badge and made me an honorary member of the United States Air Force. Sadly I lost the badge in one of my many moves since.

Military Involvement as a Surgeon

In the afternoon I went to RAF Little Rissington. They had set up there an emergency hospital consisting of ninety beds, of which twenty-two were intensive care beds fully equipped and staffed. They also had four operating tables in a row. I had assumed that I would not be allowed to photograph what I was seeing, but in fact they would have been very happy for me to photograph the amazing setup. Exactly one patient was occupying a bed. He had been involved in a local accident. Having again given my lectures and teaching, it was very apparent that Little Rissington had already decided that burn patients would be looked after at Upper Heyford. I therefore did not have to become involved in the decision.

The date for the commencement of hostilities had been decided, and was given to me and to the administration at Stoke Mandeville and Oxford, with the strict requirement that we must not divulge it. To ensure that there were beds available, all emergency surgical admissions to both hospitals stopped. However, when hostilities started, the number of casualties transferred back to England was exceptionally few, and there were no British burned military personnel needing in-patient care. After some ten days with all our empty beds and personnel with nothing to do, the senior medical officer and chief executive asked me to give permission for some normal surgical admissions to restart. With the evidence of the empty beds in front of me I had no option but to agree.

Many thousands of Iraqi soldiers and civilians were killed but only 47 British soldiers died. The Senegalese army had 92 deaths and the United States' military had a total of 149 dead. Of these 111 were killed in action, 35 in friendly fire incidents and 38 in accidents. Included in these numbers were soldiers whose sleeping accommodation and mess were hit by a SCUD missile. I was telephoned and told that these patients were coming into RAF Upper Heyford to be re-dressed and then transferred the following day to burn units in the United States. I suggested that, if it was possible, the plane should be refuelled in mid-air and flown direct to the United States, as the casualties would do much better and would be less likely to become infected outside an experienced burn unit. This was agreed, and my active involvement with the Gulf War ceased.

Conditions in the front line for medical and surgical care are often reasonable and work to improve them is continuous – but they are still not as good as established hospitals in the UK. A phtograph showing the British military tented hospital in Saudi Arabia, has been given to me by one of my ex-trainees, now Group Captain Godwin Scerri (*see* Plate 5.1).

It is interesting that although it is easily possible to find the numbers of those killed, the number of military personnel who were injured are less accessible. This is a common problem when trying to evaluate not only wars but all forms of trauma. Part of this is due to trying to define the difference between a major injury and a minor injury, and what should be included in official figures. Looking back now at the First Gulf War, the major long-term injury was from Gulf Syndrome. This caused both physical and psychiatric problems in a large number of the military who were involved in the war. It is thought that this may have been due to inhaling poison gases. It is related to myalgic encephalomyelitis/chronic fatigue syndrome, and has caused problems for a very large number of military personnel for many years afterwards.

RAF Halton is situated about 3 miles from Stoke Mandeville Hospital. This is one of the largest air force bases in Britain, and in the 1990s was mainly a basic training facility. It was also home to St Mary's Military Hospital. Founded in 1927, this was then one of several RAF hospitals in Britain. There were also RAF hospitals in Germany and in Cyprus at RAF Akrotiri. By 1990 RAF Halton was the base for the only RAF plastic surgery unit, and included a burn unit that took patients from all three services. It had been an important and famous plastic surgery unit under Air Vice Marshal Morley, and had then been commanded by Air Commodore Ronnie Brown. I had met Ronnie Brown on various occasions at plastic surgery meetings, and following the Gulf War, although he had retired, our association developed. For some time, even prior to the Gulf War, any major military burn patient sent to RAF Halton had been transferred to the Stoke Mandeville burn unit. In one of my discussions with Ronnie Brown it was suggested that the military junior trainees should come to Stoke Mandeville for burn training. After some months of these trainees attending, albeit on an irregular basis, it was agreed that they would be seconded to the NHS for six-month attachments. The first two, one RAF and one Army, started their secondment in 1991. The burn unit at Stoke Mandeville had a symbiotic relationship with RAF Halton. Patients with major burns, particularly those whose referral to a major burn unit is delayed, are likely to develop kidney failure, and need renal dialysis to have any hope of surviving. A national expert in this treatment was Air Commodore David Rainford at RAF Halton, and therefore I would send the occasional patient who needed such treatment to him at RAF Halton for their dialysis, whilst I visited them to continue their burn treatment. In return, virtually all the military burn patients were in fact sent to Stoke Mandeville.

Ronnie Brown had started his medical training at the University of Oxford, where he became President of the Oxford Union. He once showed me a photograph of former presidents taken during a reunion. Within the group there were three ex-prime ministers and several prominent politicians. I may be biased, but I think that they were privileged to be numbered with a surgeon!

Clearly this trial training was successful, and therefore for the next ten years I would have one, two or three military trainees. The majority of them came at a senior house officer level, with one at registrar level. As well as their clinical training, I tried to introduce a research project as well, and several of the trainees wrote their first medical research paper based on the treatment of burns or related topics within our department.

The majority of these attachments were successful. More than half of the trainees became plastic surgeons, and some changed their specialty during their careers. I obviously had to write a report on their period with me, and as the attachments matured I became more involved in their training. It is gratifying that at least two of the people who came to me for these attachments owe their continuing careers as plastic surgeons to me, as I was later told that my comments about them were the deciding factor for the military to continue to train them as plastic surgeons.

Unfortunately I had to give negative reports on two of the military trainees. One was quite simple in that although he was a very able surgeon, he would tell me that he could not come to the hospital the following week as the military needed him, and would then tell the military that he could not come to them as he was needed at Stoke Mandeville. Clearly both statements were untrue, and he was in fact earning money by running a locum agency for junior doctors. He was dismissed the service. The second one was much more difficult. He was extremely intelligent and very involved in research, but the problem was that he had not the judgement to differentiate between good and poor research proposals. He was also unable to take criticism. At that stage, although I had been involved in research for many years, I had only just started to supervise research and my lack of experience I think contributed to the fact that I was unable to properly support him. It turned out that I was not the only one of his consultant supervisors that had had the same problems, both with his research and with his surgical techniques. He again left the service. He later tried to sue five of us for our reports, and the case went to the High Court in London, where it was rejected. He then emigrated.

Through Mr Rodney Gunn, an ex-army orthopaedic surgeon at Milton Keynes Hospital, I would have on occasions SAS soldiers visiting to learn about burn care. When working behind enemy lines, the SAS soldiers either have learned the local language, or are competent first aiders, and therefore of use to the local population.

During my last years as a consultant I became more involved with the selection and training of military surgeons. All trainee surgeons, to continue with their training, had to be appointed at registrar level. There were a limited number of such posts throughout the country, and the military were given extra posts so that their engagement did not deplete the total number of trainees who would be expected within the NHS. At that time the postgraduate dean in surgery for the military was Surgeon Commodore Ian Jenkins of the Royal Navy. He later became a Vice Admiral and the Surgeon General of all three services. On his retirement from the Royal Navy he became the Constable and Governor of Windsor Castle. Within the NHS competition for any registrar post in plastic surgery was extremely fierce, and it was expected that any candidate, even to make the short list, would have had one or two years' previous plastic surgery experience, passed various higher exams, and/or written research papers. The minimum legal requirement, however, was six months as a plastic surgery senior house officer, and the military were trying to take advantage of this position. I had a conversation with Ian, pointing out that when we had appointed military candidates with only six months' experience behind them, they had found it extremely difficult to settle into a unit where normally the SHOs, theoretically ranked below them, had had considerably more experience. I eventually won this argument and the selection of military registrars changed. That was my first involvement in the politics of training military surgeons.

A year or two later I was appointed as the Honorary Civilian Consultant in Plastic Surgery to the Royal Air Force. This meant that as well as taking part in other discussions, I sat on, and normally chaired, various appointment committees both at consultant and at junior levels.

My next military involvement occurred through my visits to Sarajevo, both during and after the Bosnian War (*see* Chapter 6). On the first visit we flew with the Royal Canadian Air Force and then the Royal Air Force. In Sarajevo we came across both the Serbian army and also the UN military forces, particularly from Italy and France. British forces were

Military Involvement as a Surgeon

then primarily based in Banja Luka, the capital of Srpska to the north. During my second visit in October our logistician was retired Army GP Colonel John Navein. During his service he had been the GP at Hereford, the base of the SAS in Britain. UK Med, which organised the visits, was funded by the United Nations and we were therefore required to look after injured patients from both sides. This meant that on rare occasions we would go to a clinic outside the limit of the Sarajevo defence zone. Colonel Navein had contacts with the SAS personnel in Sarajevo at the time and we used to borrow their armoured Land Rover when we needed to visit the outside clinics. One evening we had a party, to which came two SAS officers and two soldiers. Home-made alcohol was very cheaply available on the roadside at 50p for a large bottle. The first two drinks were quite revolting, then for some reason further drinks became much more palatable. At the end of an excellent evening, the soldier driving their Land Rover took about seven attempts to get it moving before they drove away. The next day we went to borrow the Land Rover and was met with a somewhat frosty response from the sergeant major: 'Sorry, you can't have it today as the gentleman coming back from your party last night left it in a ditch' (although 'Gentleman' was not quite the word he used). An armoured Land Rover weighs some 4 tons and they had not yet rescued it. Happily none of the occupants was injured.

On my first visit after the war in 1996, by chance the senior surgeon at the United Nations field hospital situated just outside the city of Sarajevo was Wing Commander Godwin Scerri. He had been my first military trainee at Stoke Mandeville and we had remained in contact. I was therefore invited to go and visit him and the UN hospital. I drove there in our UN Land Rover and, having explained to the Welsh guardsmen who I was and what I was doing, they let me in unaccompanied to find Godwin. I found him playing tennis and he was astounded that I was unaccompanied as the security level of the hospital was RED at the time. It turned out that he was extremely bored and had virtually nothing to do medically and even less surgically. I suggested that he came to the University hospital to see the mine injuries we were dealing with, and to help us, particularly with a microvascular free flap that I had planned to do within the next few days. He explained that the military policy at that time was that the medical staff and hospitals were only to treat military personnel. I suggested that he should approach his commanding officer for special permission to assist me, and this was granted. I am delighted to say that the military policy has now changed. This strikes me as extremely sensible.

Plastic Surgery in Wars, Disasters and Civilian Life

Clearly military personnel have priority for treatment, but when there is time and facilities available local patients can now also be treated. This has the advantages that military people posted overseas are more welcome locally, and also the skills of the military doctors and nurses are maintained in what may be deployments lasting many months. Whether this initial decision was involved in the later change I will never know.

In 2001 I retired from the NHS and moved with my wife to the Isle of Wight. At that time military hospitals throughout Britain were closing. The Royal Hospital at Haslar was situated in Gosport, just north of the Isle of Wight. In 2001 it was still a military hospital and also looked after local civilians. It had a large plastic surgery unit staffed by Lieutenant Colonel Bennett, Wing Commander Scerri and Squadron Leader Pandya as consultants. My wife and I were invited to a reception to commemorate Armistice Day that year. When we arrived we were allocated to a junior officer who introduced us with due deference to the Surgeon General. This was Surgeon Vice Admiral Ian Jenkins, who had by then been promoted to the role. On seeing me, he put out his hand and said, 'Welcome, Anthony.' I responded with greetings to Ian. The junior officer, not knowing that we were old friends, looked considerably nonplussed. I well remember that evening, and as the final notes of the Last Post faded away at the end of the two minutes' silence, a Spitfire flew across and did a victory roll. Immaculate timing.

In 2005 Squadron Leader Pandya required sick leave and after an interview and signing the Official Secrets Act, I was asked to stand in as his locum for two days a week until his return. This was an enjoyable time. Rather than travelling every day, I stayed in a cabin in Fort Blockhouse and lived and ate in the officers' mess (wardroom). I also became involved in teaching the junior staff and in particular two of them who were preparing for the MRCS exam. I was still examining it at the time, and I am pleased to say that my two candidates both passed. The other thing that I remember about this period is being told after my six months that I was the only locum who had not left any surgical complications.

Haslar Hospital (*see* Plates 5.2 and 5.3) has a very interesting history. The Admiralty acquired the site in 1745. The hospital was designed by Theodore Jacobsen and when completed would have been the largest brick building in Europe. Construction of the main building, known as the Royal Hospital Haslar, was completed in 1762, but patients had been admitted from 1753. The original design was for 350 patients. It was built on a peninsula, and the guard towers, high brick walls, bars and railings throughout the site were all designed to prevent patients, many of whom had been press-ganged, from going AWOL (Absent Without Official Leave). The hospital also included an asylum for sailors with psychiatric disorders.

Amongst the notable doctors who have worked there is Dr James Lind (1716–1794), a leading physician at Haslar from 1758 till 1785. He played a major part in discovering a cure for scurvy, through his pioneering use of a double-blind methodology with Vitamin C supplements (limes). The hospital also established the country's first blood bank and treated casualties from the Normandy landings in 1944. It was renamed the Royal Naval Hospital Haslar in 1954 to reflect its naval traditions. A tri-military burn unit was built and opened in the hospital in 1996. For a reason that I have never understood it was closed on the same day that it was officially opened, and burn casualties from the military continued to be treated in NHS hospitals.

The hospital's remit became tri-service in 1996 when it reverted to being called the Royal Hospital, Haslar. A hyperbaric medicine unit was established at the hospital at that time particularly for the treatment of divers and submariners. The hospital was handed over to the NHS in 2007 and was closed in 2009 when the staff and patients were transferred to Queen Alexandra's Hospital in Portsmouth.

I found Haslar to be of the most friendly hospitals in which I have ever worked. This was partly due to its relatively small size and the numbers of patients and staff, but also because the nursing staff, who were mostly military, were excellent and reminded me of the nurses of thirty years before. The hospital itself, although 250 years old, was spotless and had almost the lowest rate of MRSA infection in the country. Just 3 miles away the hospital in Portsmouth had one of the highest rates. Again because of the small numbers, I became friends with several of the consultants in other specialties, and I would regularly go to watch them, and occasionally assist, in the operating theatres. I particularly got to know Air Commodore Bryan Morgans, who at that time was head of general surgery for the tri-services. He very kindly proposed me, and Air Commodore Brown seconded me, for the Royal Air Force Club in Piccadilly. I was elected as an associate member, and I both stayed in the club and ate there fairly regularly when in London. It was by far the best and cheapest restaurant that I came across in the City. I resigned from the club last year as I was no longer using it, and what had been a very cheap annual subscription was slowly creeping up. Whilst at Haslar, I also became a member of the Fort

Blockhouse Officers' Mess. As well as living there, there were special annual occasions to celebrate events such as the Battle of Trafalgar, the Battle of Waterloo, Burns night and the Battle of Britain. These were held with full pageantry, in uniform or dinner jackets, and with a military quartet playing in the gallery. An occasion that I particularly remember was a Battle of Britain display, and afterwards the Red Arrows pilots came to the mess for tea. Quite rightly the pilots were very proud of themselves, but this was obviously an excuse for 'taking the Michael'. They were known by their numbers, and as one introduced himself as Red 3, he was met with the comment, 'I didn't know that the Royal Air Force was staffed by communists.' I don't think he was amused.

I was also in contact with the commanding officer of the Hospital, Surgeon Captain James Campbell, who later invited me to conferences to lecture about my experience of wars and disasters. The third person with whom I became friendly was the second-in-command, Rear Admiral Lionel Jervis. He later became the Prior of St John, where again we came into contact. My regret at not being in the services returned, and I was particularly sad that I was not eligible for overseas service, either in Afghanistan or in the Ebola crisis, to which my military personnel colleagues were posted.

During the time of my involvement with the military there had been major changes. In the beginning the three services had distinct medical services, with all of the specialties being catered for in each service. Over the years this changed. When a doctor signed up for the services, they would join either the Army, the navy or the RAF, as junior doctors still do, and would spend a period of between six months and three years doing basic medical care (in effect, general practice) within that service. During this period, possibly by inclination but also by selection, they could be appointed to a training scheme in a specialty. I have already talked about the problems of the military extra numbers and the solution to it. All training of junior doctors at this level in the services is now within the NHS, and I hope that this was partly caused by my arguments with the then future Surgeon General.

The other change that has occurred is that at consultant level, again in all specialties, military medical care is now theoretically tri-service. However, this has not completely happened and each service still has a number of posts within each specialty. It became ridiculous some years ago when a colleague of mine who was a paediatrician and Surgeon Captain in the Navy was invited to change to the Army and be promoted to the rank of brigadier. He would have done the same job, but declined the offer and retired from the services. I completely failed to see the logic of the situation. As the military numbers in all three services have declined, so the numbers of doctors, nurses and other military staff have of course reduced too. Completely illogically, the military also reduced the highest level of promotion that a doctor could reach as a clinician. When I was first involved this was air commodore in the RAF but became group captain. I know this severely affected one of my friends who was about to be appointed air commodore when the system changed.

The other major change has been caused by the loss of military hospitals, and what happens now at consultant level is that all military personnel are attached to an NHS hospital, but on the condition that they can be posted overseas at any time if required. There are two major hospitals in use. Queen Elizabeth Hospital in Birmingham, which has now taken over from Selly Oak Hospital, is the major military centre. The original plan was to build this in Oxford, but unfortunately there was insufficient room on the site of the John Radcliffe Hospital. Had that happened, then Stoke Mandeville Hospital would have been the burn and spinal injuries centre. The Navy uses Derriford Hospital in Plymouth. The Royal Air Force does not have one particular hospital, although the largest plastic surgery unit is in Portsmouth.

In 2001, much to my surprise, it was suggested by Air Commodore Morgans that I take a locum post as the consultant general surgeon at RAF Akrotiri in Cyprus to cover the vacation of Colonel Muri Ismaeli. Colonel Ismaeli had been the resident military general surgeon in Cyprus for several years and clearly enjoyed the posting there with his wife. He was a remarkable man. After his retirement, he spent some time helping the victims of a major earthquake in the north of his native Pakistan. When I met him afterwards, he said that when he was operating on the victims, he had wished that he had had some training in plastic surgery. All British military surgeons now do have some training in plastic surgery and burns.

This offer of a locum position was a surprise to me, and nowadays would be even more of a surprise as the post was in a different specialty from that in which I was registered. However, in my training we had all spent three years doing general surgery, and I had been a locum senior registrar in general surgery at a major London hospital. I did, in fact, feel that it would be more appropriate for me to go as a consultant surgeon rather than as a consultant general surgeon. I went then, and twice subsequently, to Princess Mary's Hospital, situated about a mile from the main base and officers' mess at RAF Akrotiri. The flight out was in various planes, including an ancient VC 10 from RAF Brize Norton. The first time I went I was with an RAF officer who explained that I was an honorary air commodore, and I was therefore offered a VIP room in the Gateway Hotel. This was the considerably flattering name of the very modest accommodation in the base. I was also offered special seating and a visit to the flight deck on the plane. It is interesting that all the passenger seats on military planes face to the rear, a very obvious precaution to reduce casualties in the event of an accident. The duties in the hospital entailed general surgical clinics and operating lists, which I selected to fit my skills. I became an expert at doing vasectomies, which I had not done for several years. In Cyprus there were major military surgical emergencies only two or three times a year, normally following accidents. I rapidly acquired the reputation of always being there when these emergencies occurred. I remember two particularly unfortunate road traffic accidents. Although the worst casualty survived his initial treatment, he was then flown back to England where he died. I also remember using my Zambian-learned method of reducing a dislocated hip in a young lad who had been playing soccer.

Once a week I had to drive to the army base at Dhekelia at the other end of the island to do a clinic. I certainly found the mess there far less friendly than the RAF mess, but at least it was a pleasant day away from the hospital. The other thing I noticed when doing clinics anywhere was that even when they were not in uniform, I could tell within a few minutes whether they were Army or Air Force personnel. They were enjoyable times, but as I was unfortunately the only general surgeon on site, I was on 24-hour cover. This meant that I could not easily go sailing, but I did have several training flights as I could always come down rapidly onto the airfield if required. And the birdwatching and the go-karting were both top class.

It was an excellent and friendly mess in which United States Air Force (USAF) personnel were present in some numbers. USAF messes are dry (no alcohol), and this accounted for the presence of the American officers in our mess. We obviously knew what they were doing at RAF Akrotiri as we were looking after them medically, but could not discuss their military role outside the air base. Two other things happened whilst I was there. The first was 9/11, the attack on the World Trade Centre in New York. This put up the security level to RED and grounded all planes for several days. The second thing that happened was that preparations were being

Military Involvement as a Surgeon

made for the Second Gulf War, and the commander of the naval helicopter squadron that was passing through Akrotiri was a marine, Major Marcus Chandler. He was a friend and neighbour from the Isle of Wight. He organised for me to have a flight around Cyprus in a naval helicopter, which was interesting on two fronts. Firstly it turned out later that no one over the age of 60 is allowed to fly in a military helicopter. Somehow this was ignored. The second thing was that the flight provided some practice for the aircrew at navigating without GPS. They were, in fact, not very good at this. They would look at the map in some puzzlement, and I would suggest that I could see a lake below. They would then ask which lake I thought it was. It turned out that I did most of the navigating.

Princess Mary's Hospital closed in 2013 and was demolished in 2016.

After these working visits to Cyprus I became a member of the Military Surgical Society and went to their meetings both in England and also in Cyprus and in Gibraltar. I presented papers at all of these and was able to renew friendships from the past and to make new ones. I was also made a member of the Combined Services Plastic Surgery Society, and I have been to, and still attend, several of their meetings around Britain. It is a chance to see how my old trainees and colleagues have been progressing in their careers, and to keep up with changes in plastic surgery in the military.

In 2008 my wife and I visited our daughter and son-in-law at the British Army Training Unit Suffield (BATUS) in Alberta, Canada. At that time our son-in-law, Major Paul Feenan, was commanding the helicopter squadron at the camp. The camp covers an area in Alberta larger than Wales. It exists for live firing exercises for members of the British Army, who go there for short detachments. Again there were rules for helicopter flying – pilots could not fly their own families, and the over-60 rule again applied – but these were luckily not thought to apply to us, and we had a very pleasant flight, skippered by Paul, around the area to see its vastness and wilderness.

Probably my last formal involvement with the military, except for conferences, came during my disaster work in the Philippines following the typhoon of 2013. My half of the relief team was based on the destroyer HMS *Daring* – or as the BBC called it on one occasion HMS *Darling* – which we thought somewhat unfortunate for the navy. We lived in cabins and in the wardroom (the naval officers' mess). The ship moved through the islands to the north of Cebu and we used the helicopter to fly to two or three islands each day to assess the damage and to see what was required in the way of medical care. By the time we got to some of these islands it was several days after the typhoon and there was virtually no care needed in the clinics apart from re-dressings and assessments of the damage. Again the rule of flying in helicopters over 60 was luckily ignored.

Thoughts and Summary

Having often become involved with the military in my career I think that I would have enjoyed a military career. However, as I said earlier, the great problem of being in the military is that to a very large extent one's choices regarding one's career path can be contrary to the wishes or experience of the person. I have found that there is often a happy and supportive attitude within many, if not most, NHS messes, but it is nothing to that found in military messes. There are clearly problems within the military – perhaps the most obvious that I noticed was the lack of secretarial help, and with the amount of paperwork that the military require, this was a great handicap. But this would have been vastly overset by the backing and help of the administration and logisticians, which I valued on several occasions. Certainly when I was working at Haslar, if I asked for a piece of equipment or help, I know not how but it was found by the next day. If only that had been the case in the NHS.

In conclusion, I have enormous respect for the military medical services and for those who work within them.

Chapter 6

Medical Care in Disasters and Wars

Disasters

The *Oxford English Dictionary* defines a disaster as 'An unfavourable aspect of a star or planet' or 'Anything that befalls of a ruinous or distressing nature; a sudden or great misfortune, mishap, or misadventure; a calamity.' For a child, losing a toy is a disaster; for a teenager, being rejected by a boy or girlfriend is a disaster; for an adult, losing one's husband or wife is a disaster. And everyone would agree that the Lockerbie air crash of 1988, when 270 people in the plane and 11 residents hit by falling debris were killed, was a disaster. At Lockerbie a few people on the ground also received minor injuries, and these were easily treated locally. But none of the above is a medical disaster.

So what is a medical disaster? It is surprisingly difficult to define, but a reasonable definition is a situation when there are more injured patients than can be treated locally. Dead patients are not included as they do not need treatment. This definition means that there can be very different numbers of patients involved. For example, on a small Scottish island two or three major injuries might be a disaster, whereas in the centre of a large city a major hospital could manage six such patients without a problem.

I have divided medical disasters into various categories, and have found this useful when lecturing around the world:

- Level D1: Patients can be treated at the local hospital, but may require additional staff to be called in;
- Level D2: Patients can be treated at several hospitals within the region;
- Level D3: Patients can be treated within a country;
- Level D4: International help is required; and
- Level D5: Unmanageable – there are too many injured patients to be treated. An example of the D5 category was the Haiti earthquake.

Disasters can also be separated into natural and man-made disasters:

	Deaths	Injuries	Situation*	Destruction
Natural				
Earthquake	High	High	Poor	Severe
Volcano	Moderate	Moderate	Poor	High
Forest Fires	Low	Moderate	Poor	Severe
Floods	Low	Very low	Moderate	High
Tsunami	High	Low	Moderate	Severe
Typhoons	Low	Moderate	Poor	Very severe
Man-Made				
Land Transport	High	High	Moderate	Low
Air Transport	High	Low	Moderate	Low
Building Fires	Moderate	Low	Good	Moderate
Terrorism	High	High	Good	Moderate
Explosions	High	High	Moderate	Moderate

* Situation refers to the proximity of first aid and hospitals.

Most doctors, nurses and paramedics will not be involved in a medical disaster during their whole career. It is more common among military staff, orthopaedic and plastic and burn surgeons, but still unlikely.

Medical disasters are normally well described in the medical literature. However, searches of disasters as reported by the non-medical press are frequently inconclusive as deaths are reported, but not injuries. One problem in reporting injuries is the degree of severity, and whether, for instance, a minor bruise should be included. This problem is compounded if, as happens, a country or body wishes to make the incident appear more or less severe. At least dead bodies are definable.

I am one of the 'unlikely' doctors. Whilst training at the Birmingham Accident Hospital I looked after one of the Birmingham Bombing victims and also two patients transferred from the Libyan War. These came to me some time after their injuries had occurred. My real involvement with disaster medicine started with the Bradford stadium fire, which happened in May 1985, when I had been appointed as a consultant at Stoke Mandeville Hospital and was working my three months' notice in Bradford.

Bradford Football Stadium Fire, 11 May 1985

Bradford FC had just been promoted to Division 2 and were playing the final game of the season against Lincoln FC. The ground and the stadium were full of fans celebrating the promotion, and the match was being televised live. At 3.40pm smoke was noticed coming from the upper part of the old wooden stadium (*see* Plate 6.1). Four and a half minutes later (Plate 6.2) many people had been burned, a large number of them severely.

Neither David Sharpe, the consultant on call, nor I were called by the hospital. This was before the days of mobile phones and the hospital bleepers only worked within the hospital. The staff had been able to bleep our resident senior house officer, Dr Mossad, but could not mobilise the full team because incoming calls to the hospital had priority over outgoing calls, and as the match was being televised, a large number of people were phoning in to enquire about their relatives. About thirty minutes after the fire broke out, I was watching the news on television and saw the reports of the fire. I put the flashing light on my car and drove to the Bradford Royal Infirmary. To any young doctor now it would be quite amazing that there were no specialised consultants in casualty, and the higher level of care was given by consultant orthopaedic surgeons (orthopods), normally on a daily rotation. Orthopaedic surgeons have, I think, never quite understood the importance of plastic surgeons in managing trauma, but the look of relief on the face of the consultant who was there when I arrived will remain with me. The whole of the casualty department and the surrounding corridors were full of badly burned and mostly elderly patients, and ambulances were still arriving. There were five patients with orthopaedic problems and the orthopod took over their care; the anaesthetists took over the care of the patients with breathing problems; and I took over the rest, with help from Dr Mossad, who had had burn experience in Egypt before he came to us and had been doing well.

The order of priorities for the initial assessment of a burned patient is firstly, their ability to breathe: facial burns and smoke inhalation can affect this severely, and can cause early death. The second priority is the extent of the burn. This is measured as a percentage of the total skin area that is burned. Although taught in medical school, without experience it is normally grossly overestimated. If the area burned is more than 15 per cent of the skin total area in an adult, then intravenous fluid is ideally required. The third priority is covering the burn. In addition, it can be very important that any associated major injury is found and treated, as often that may need even more rapid treatment than the burn. Throughout these stages pain relief and reassurance are crucial. With experience, the first two critical stages can be done in about one minute, but writing it down, which is of course essential, takes far longer. If there is one patient this is obviously no problem, but with fifty patients time becomes critical. On the spot I devised the method of tape recording my findings and after every five patients the tapes were taken away by a series of secretaries for typing. The situation was complicated as the plastic surgery unit with specialised nurses and beds was at St Luke's Hospital about 1½ miles away. The nurses in particular were needed for dressing the burns, which takes far longer than the assessments.

At about 7.30pm David Sharpe, the plastic surgery consultant on call (and in fact the only one in Bradford at that time, as his colleague Mr Crocket was on leave) arrived looking somewhat flustered. He had learned about the fire when the local private hospital had phoned David with the message, 'When you have time from the disaster, could you come and see a burned patient who had arrived for private treatment?'

David and I had been friends and colleagues for many years. We had been appointed senior registrars at the same interview five years previously, and he had taken the consultant post in Bradford when Mr Tom Barclay had retired. Ironically he had taken that post because he did not want burns as a major part of his job. I had not applied because I did want burn care to be part of my future work.

David was a good manager, and rapidly became a very experienced one. In discussion with the management in both hospitals, it was decided that a ward could be emptied at St Luke's Hospital and anyone who needed admission could be moved there. This had several advantages: patients did not have to be moved to other hospitals with burn units that were many miles away, and being together the patients were able to help each other psychologically, as well as being able to be visited by relatives. Three children with burns were also moved to the paediatric ward at St Luke's.

All of the patients who needed admission were moved to St Luke's overnight. There were twenty-one patients requiring intravenous resuscitation, and another fifteen or so who clearly needed surgery. There were five with other medical problems, four orthopaedic injuries as their main problem, one child with a head injury and four adults with smoke inhalation. One of these I well remember. When first seen in casualty he was blue and appeared to be breathing his last. We all thought his chances of survival were zero and he was given oxygen and nursing care only. Three days later, quite unbelievably, he came round, and his very first words were, 'When can I have a smoke?' I managed to refrain from answering.

At the first selection of patients at the fire, ten of the most severely burned patients had been sent by the ambulance teams to Pinderfields

Hospital in Wakefield. This was the regional burn unit for Yorkshire, where the very experienced consultant was Dr John Settle. Several of those ten patients, because of their age and burn severity, had no chance of survival, but nevertheless were occupying intensive care beds. Although it sounds unsympathetic, these patients should have been nursed in side-rooms until their death, leaving the intensive care beds for those who had a chance of survival and really needed them.

In trying to escape the fire, some spectators dropped down some 6 feet over the wall at the front of the stand, causing a few injuries. Very fortunately there was no barrier of the sort which in 1989 caused so many of the ninety-six deaths at the Hillsborough stadium disaster in Sheffield. At Bradford it was thought that only one patient had died at the time, but when the inferno had died down that night it was found that many of the spectators had tried to escape down stairways leading to emergency doors. Tragically these doors were locked to prevent unlawful entry. Some were broken down, but some were not, and about fifty bodies were found.

The next morning we did a ward round to talk to the patients and to work out what surgery was required, and what was possible in Bradford. After a discussion, it was agreed that by bringing in surgeons and other staff from other hospitals, all the necessary surgery could be done at St Luke's. David then went off with the management to work out how this was to be done, and then phoned the necessary colleagues, who were all able to put off other responsibilities and come to help on a rota basis. What astonished us was the rapidity of the arrival of the press – first nationally, and then internationally. We calculated that within a few days there were more press than patients, in total over two hundred people. We had at that time no experience or training in dealing with the press, but David in particular, and I to a lesser extent, soon learned.

We knew that there were other people who had been burned, but the extent of their burns did not require urgent admission. It was announced on the radio that there would be a clinic on the Monday, and I was asked to take two of the junior staff to the Bradford Royal Infirmary to organise it. Again, there was disbelief when more than 150 patients appeared, mostly with minor burns, but several with deep, although not extensive, burns, which would be better treated with early surgery. The planned 2-hour clinic went on for most of the day, and at the end another fifteen or so patients had to be added to the list for operations and arrangements made for their admission. Then followed my first experience with the press. I was interviewed for the BBC by Kate Adie, who was absolutely delightful, put me at ease, and asked no awkward questions. A few days later I did one further interview with Anne Diamond for ITV, which was much less satisfactory. It was in a studio talking to a television screen in the early hours of the morning, which was less than friendly as I had been operating solidly for the previous two days. And to finish, she asked the usual question which happens in so many interviews – 'Have the patients been upset by their experience?' or similar wording. It is difficult to answer without being rude and saying what a stupid question.

And then we operated every day for more than two weeks. There were no major problems, and although some were at risk, none of the patients at St Luke's Hospital died.

The fire was a national event and widely covered by both the national and international press. And, of course, we had visitors. Prince Charles visited Wakefield, and Mr and Mrs Thatcher and Mr and Mrs Kinnock visited Bradford. One of the major problems of burn care is infection. This was explained to Mrs Thatcher, who immediately agreed that she would visit the ward with no press, and not shake any patient's hand. I did shake her hand and commented that she had Dupuytren's disease. Her response was, 'How do you know?' Since I had just been appointed a consultant hand surgeon the answer was rather obvious! In fact she went into a ward full of mostly elderly Yorkshiremen, who were, I think, mostly Labour supporters, but she came out from a ward full of Tory supporters! She was marvellous. During the afternoon I was detailed to look after Mr Denis Thatcher. This was not an easy job as his dementia was starting. When Mr Kinnock came, the same worries about infection were explained to him, but he was unhappy without the press attending, although with prompting he managed not to shake any patient's hands. I was given Mrs Kinnock to look after, which was a much easier job. She was a very impressive lady. She was particularly keen on seeing our one remaining child with his head injury, which had occurred when he fell over the stand wall, and she then talked to all the other children on the paediatric ward. The third interesting visit was from Robert Maxwell, who came with his team to present a cheque. It turned out the cheque was from his readers and not his own money, but it was welcome anyway. He was a very large man in all ways, and I noticed that one of his senior staff was trembling when Maxwell was speaking to him. The reporters from his newspapers were with him, and David said to Maxwell that he was worried about the accuracy of what they would report. Maxwell turned to his reporters and said that nothing was to be published until it had been checked. David then appointed me as the checker, which was somewhat annoying as they were to phone me at about 3.00am for several days for the checking. Interestingly the reporters were then attached to us for some days and they did say that they had never been given the same instruction before. Very little did in fact need correcting, and it was mostly medical terms.

One problem that did arise was the lack of trained plastic surgery nurses to do the first dressings. This had not been foreseen, and other nurses had to be brought in. All of the patients had been interviewed by a psychiatrist during their stay. This was the first time that this had been done after a disaster, at least in the UK, with the aim of reducing post-traumatic stress disorder (PTSD). In clinics afterwards the general feeling from the patients was that the fact they had been kept together had given them a chance to discuss their problems, and that had been much more useful than the psychiatric sessions. David had made the very sensible decision that rather than discharging the patients in dribs and drabs, they would be sent home almost together after three weeks when most were well on their way to being healed, and this had also helped.

At the end of the three weeks David was asked in one interview what had been new about the incident. The answers were the facts that the fire had been televised, and that the patients had been kept together rather than distributed around several hospitals. When pushed, he also mentioned the 'Bradford Sling', which he had developed some time earlier to elevate burned (or otherwise injured) hands and the superglue 'Histoacryl', which was used to stick skin grafts in place. I had done the early research on the latter and published it in 1976. It had been used occasionally since then, but after the interview both David's sling and the use of superglue have spread around the world and are now standard procedures.

Although most of the work was done in Bradford and Wakefield, eight inpatients and forty-eight outpatients were treated in other hospitals.

In October 1985 a panel discussion was organised in Bradford with the support of the Smith & Nephew Foundation. Twenty-three doctors, nurses, ambulance personnel and managers met to discuss the outcomes of the disaster and the lessons to be learned. The results were published by the Royal Society of Medicine (*see* References). The conclusions were that keeping patients together had been important; that the initial sorting at the scene of the disaster should have been done by experienced plastic surgery consultants, and that specialist nurses should be imported. It also noted that the telephone systems in hospitals should be changed so that an outgoing line would always be available.

The follow-up of the disaster included the Popplewell Enquiry, the setting-up of a research fund by David Sharpe, and subsequently awards of OBEs to David Sharpe and John Settle, and an MBE to the Matron.

For me personally, it marked the start of my international work around the world. I was asked to present a paper at the International Society of Burn Injuries in Australia and my visit was funded by Smith & Nephew, and then went to South Africa the following year. I am also sure that my work in disasters and wars was a major contribution to the OBE that I was later awarded.

In 2015 a book was published by Martin Fletcher entitled 'Fifty-six: The Story of the Bradford Fire'. It includes several criticisms, particularly of the Popplewell Enquiry.

Athens Oil Refinery Fire, 1 September 1992

In September 1992 I received a phone call from Dr Lochaitis, a Greek plastic surgeon whom I had met at a number of conferences, asking me if it was possible to bring out a team to help with patients injured during an explosion and fire that had occurred at the Elefsina Oil Refinery 10 miles from Athens. We quickly sorted out details about travel, accommodation and money, all funded by the owner of the refinery. I recruited my senior registrar, Rob Ratcliffe, Sister Sue Fox from our burn unit, and two junior surgical trainees from Mount Vernon Hospital burn unit. The team was flown by private plane from Luton Airport, and with an incredibly rapid passage arranged through immigration and customs we arrived in Athens and that afternoon we visited three hospitals to assess the extent of the injuries. It became apparent that all of the seventeen or eighteen patients occupying the intensive care beds had burns of 90 per cent or more, which in adults is not survivable. There were also other patients with lesser burns, who should have been in those beds. I did an interview on Greek national television, and confirmed that 'Wherever they were treated in the world, there was sadly no chance of these severely injured patients surviving.' Dr Lochaitis thanked me profusely and said that if he had said that, no one would have believed him. This was my discovery of the power of an international opinion. I then spent the rest of the night in the best suite in the best hotel in Athens, but I do not remember eating. The next day we visited the remaining hospitals with intensive care patients who were in the same situation.

The unsurvivable burn patient, if not given intravenous fluid, will die within a few hours. If they are treated with fluids, antibiotics, ventilation, etc., then they can survive for some days. In fact the last of the patients whom we had seen in Athens survived for four weeks. The problem occurs when one of these patients is admitted to an intensive care bed, as it is unacceptable to relatives and to others for them to be taken elsewhere in the hospital to die. This is an argument that I have faced around the world. The counter-argument that people use is that the patients are no longer being treated properly unless they are in intensive care. This is not true: they are being properly treated but in an ordinary bed, ideally in a side ward, with pain relief, no painful procedures and with someone to talk to until they lose consciousness and die. They will endure no further painful procedures. And this way the intensive care bed can be used for a patient who does have a chance of survival. Similar decisions have had to be made with Covid. These must have been far more difficult to make, as we know and can measure the survival chances in a burned patient, but the research on Covid patient survival chances has still to be done.

After further discussion and telephone calls, it was agreed that four of the seriously injured, but possibly survivable patients, would be flown to England, two to Stoke Mandeville and two to Mount Vernon. This was organised in a commercial airliner, which was less than ideal as simple things such as arranging four beds, safety belts and suspending intravenous bottles of fluid were not simple. But manage we did, and Plate 6.3 shows the result. We landed back at Luton and the four patients were transferred, two to Mount Vernon by helicopter and two to Stoke Mandeville by ambulance. The ambulance with blue lights flashing went through red traffic lights when necessary, and I had to follow in my car with my green flashing light and hand on the horn, but without a problem.

The two patients at Stoke Mandeville were already infected, only two days after the fire, and tragically the older and more severely burned patient died. This also happened at Mount Vernon.

Overall there were twenty deaths and twenty-one survivors, many of whom would have required further surgery.

We had the thanks of Dr Lochaitis and of the refinery owner. I suggested that instead of me sending an invoice for my services, he should contribute to our research fund. I am still waiting.

The Hong Kong Mountain Disaster, 10 February 1996

In 1996 I was visiting Hong Kong for an International Surgical Conference. Also at this conference was Colonel Basil Pruitt, who was the senior burn surgeon and researcher in the United States. We had met several times previously at conferences around the world and had become friends, although we always argued about the most appropriate fluid for resuscitation in burn patients.

While the conference was taking place, a fire had broken out in dry forest at Pat Sin Leng mountain reserve in the New Territories. A school party hiking there had got caught up in it. Basil and I were asked by Professor Walter King of the Chinese University of Hong Kong, who was the consultant looking after the survivors, to visit the patients in the burn unit at the Prince of Wales Hospital in Sha Tin and offer advice. There were seven severely burned children, three of whom had been paralysed and put on respirators. They were being well managed, and our contributions were minimal. Overall, three students and two teachers died at the scene, and of the seven injured, one died in hospital.

About a year later I was asked to do a medico-legal examination of two of the students, although it was later decided that as I had seen them whilst they were being treated, it would be inappropriate for me to do so. What had happened was that when they were in intensive care, paralysed and unconscious, an excess of the fluid that was being used to replace their losses built up in their legs. This is known as Compartment Syndrome, and in a conscious patient is extremely painful, making it easy to diagnose. An unconscious patient would of course be unaware of the problem. The increased pressure causes severe wasting of the muscles and nerves unless released, and that is what had happened to the two boys, causing permanent, and very difficult to treat, injuries.

Basil and I had disagreed at several meetings about the most appropriate fluid to be used in resuscitation in burn units. He believed in electrolytes and I in colloids. Both have problems, but in the paralysed patient electrolytes, which had been used in the Hong Kong patients, were more dangerous.

Colonel Basil Pruitt died in 2019 at the age of 88, and it is still my regret that I had not visited him at Fort Sam Houston in the United States.

The Haiti Earthquake, 12 January 2010

At 4.53pm in the afternoon of 12 January 2010 an earthquake of magnitude 7.0 occurred 25km west of the centre of Port au Prince, the capital of the Republic of Haiti. It was relatively close to the surface and therefore caused very severe damage and loss of life. Many thousands of people were killed and injured, and very many more were trapped in collapsed buildings. It was obvious almost from the beginning that this was a D5 level disaster. Fortunately, although the main hospital had been damaged, it was still functioning. It would, however, have reached its capacity very rapidly. As the port and the airport had both been badly damaged and were not usable, the only ingress into the country at the beginning was via a poor mountainous road from the neighbouring Dominican Republic. The border was 30 miles away, and the capital and major hospital in Santo Domingo were 160 miles away. Very soon teams from countries around the world offered assistance. The first international help came from the Dominican Republic, the Cuban Government and the US Navy Hospital Ship *Comfort*. Repairs to the docks and airport were arranged internationally. Eventually fourteen countries and 135 Non-Governmental Organisations (NGOs) arrived to help, often by erecting and staffing field hospitals.

The British response was organised by Medical Emergency Relief International (MERLIN). As well as their own staff, and with the aid of various professional societies, including the British Association of Plastic Surgeons, the British Orthopaedic Association and the Anaesthetic Association, the necessary specialists required to staff a reconstructive hospital were recruited. A tented hospital was set up in the grounds of a local tennis club and was appropriately named the Wimbledon Hospital (*see* Plate 6.4). Local nursing, security and other staff were hired, and living accommodation and transport were also arranged.

It was obvious from the beginning that relatively long-term help would be needed, and therefore the British consultants and nurses organised themselves into a rota. I was to be in the final group that went out, ten weeks after the earthquake. An orthopaedic surgeon and one anaesthetist were staying out there on an extended basis (Plate 6.5), and I and the second anaesthetist flew from London to Santo Domingo, and then by a UN flight to Port au Prince. I took over from Mr Remo Papini, a plastic surgeon from Birmingham, who handed his patients over to me before flying home. After his arrival in London he suffered a severe pulmonary embolus when a blood clot moved from his leg into his lungs. Very luckily he survived. Talking to some of the earlier teams months later, it was clear that they had found life stressful, with a large number of patients needing urgent treatment, and even more so as the hospital had not been fully constructed.

When I was there, the majority of the patients were in the middle of their treatment, or were coming for further surgery. There was still the occasional patient from the quake coming in having had no previous treatment. I remember one young girl who had a severely deformed hand with poor function. We had an X-ray machine available, and the X-ray showed multiple fractures of her hand and fingers. About ten weeks after the injury, these had almost healed. Surgery would have been possible, but it would have required a series of operations and physiotherapy over a year or two. I was in the last team, so this would not be possible, and sadly I had to tell her that there was nothing that could be done. The other surgery that the orthopaedic surgeon and I were doing came about because of a connection with a hospital which the American charity Heartline had occupied (see Plate 6.6). It was being used primarily for medical patients and there were no surgical facilities or staff. The nursing was excellent, and they had a physiotherapist and a local psychologist. When our beds were full, they would take our patients for post-operative nursing, and in return we would operate on their patients as needed. The lack of a physiotherapist in the Wimbledon Hospital caused some problems, particularly for the many patients who had lost one or more limbs. An arrangement was made with the charity Handicap International, whose staff came in on most days to offer their help and to fit artificial limbs when required. Because many patients had been trapped in falling buildings, there had been a large number who had had to have limbs amputated, causing an unusual casualty situation.

The nursing was a mixture of our nurses and local nurses, and the standard was good. MERLIN had also employed a local medical student as a translator. He rapidly reverted to being a medical student as well, and he was delightful and able. When we left he thanked us profusely and commented very favourably on the teaching he had received. He also had a brother who had somehow managed to acquire a fresh small cut on his face. It clearly needed suturing. He thought that if I, a plastic surgeon, sewed him up, then there would be no scar. I had to disillusion him before the operation, and he was very upset.

And so for two weeks whatever surgery was needed we did. The hospital was also running a very busy out-patient facility which anybody could attend, whether from the quake or for any other medical reason. I was often called by the doctor running it to see a patient, and one that I well remember had a leaking wound and several lumps on the side of her neck. Our British out-patient doctor, not surprisingly, was baffled by the diagnosis of what is now a very rare condition in the UK. I instantly recognised cervical tuberculosis (TB), which I had not seen since I had had the same condition more than sixty years earlier. The patient was sent off to the

Government hospital for medical treatment. The clinic had several patients who needed surgery which I could easily have done, but the policy of MERLIN, or at least the junior doctor who was in charge of us, said that we could only operate on victims of the quake. This was unfortunate, and upset me considerably, as there was spare time and the facilities were available.

There were other problems, too. Certainly the high temperature was one. The only tent that was air-conditioned was the operating theatre and that made operating much more enjoyable. The other problem was moving between our residence and the hospital or anywhere else. We had to be in a small coach in radio contact with our base. This was completely understandable because of an earlier kidnap of relief workers. Being in the coach made photography much more difficult, particularly as we had been advised to only take small cameras so as not to upset people. My new camera was very slow to focus compared to my usual Nikon, and as the coach was normally moving, the results were less than perfect. There had been worries about photographing people and patients. In fact everyone appeared to enjoy having their photograph taken, particularly when they were shown their image on the screen of the camera.

We did have one day off, when we drove to a local tourist area with an old castle. There we got out of the coach and walked around, and enjoyed an excellent packed lunch. On the way back a very large house was pointed out to us. This was the home of the voodoo priest, a very important person in an area where voodooism was still common, and in fact almost universal even amongst Christian communities.

There was other work also happening in the hospital as ShelterBoxes were being made up. When a patient was discharged, they were given one of these boxes containing food and basic necessities to tide them over the next few days wherever they were going to stay (Plate 6.7). This was often to be in a tented camp.

Although I had seen earthquake damage before, it was never on the same scale (Plate 6.8). In terms of the power of the quake, it was a thousand times less powerful at 7.0 on the logarithmic scale than the most powerful ever recorded at 10. However, on the mortality scale it was somewhere around the fourth most disastrous in recorded history, with more than 250,000 people dead, as well as more than 300,000 injured and 500,000 displaced. What made this so severe was that the epicentre was close to a large city with many poorly constructed buildings. I noticed when being driven around that buildings of wooden construction, which could shake, had very often survived. The quake occurred in one of the poorest countries in the world, where rescue and medical services were desperately poor compared to many other countries, and this increased both the death and the long-term injury rates.

In my previous experiences of disasters, funding had been provided either by the government or by specific donations. I found it very difficult to accept that MERLIN had as many people on site involved in publicity and fund-raising as there were clinical workers. I realise that charities need to raise money, but that situation I thought was over the top.

On my return, I was asked to write a report. The recruiting of surgeons, anaesthetists and nurses working through our professional bodies was simple and effective. The tented hospital and the accommodation were more than adequate under the conditions. Having always to be in a vehicle when moving around was frustrating, but as two relief workers from another charity had been kidnapped only two weeks previously, it was completely understandable. (Both were later released unharmed and with no ransom paid.) The multiple briefings were, however, repetitive and the evening meetings not useful. Had a clinical member of the resident staff been on the morning ward rounds as requested, this would have been very useful in planning. Of far greater use would have been a computer in theatre and secretarial help with the clinical notes, which were often very poor. My main complaint was that a very junior doctor, although delightful, was in overall control, and telling senior consultants what they could or could not do. With her lack of experience, this caused frustration as it would have been perfectly possible to have done other useful surgery when there were no quake victims needing help. Far better for the role would have been an experienced and perhaps retired senior consultant.

Another problem which upset many of my military colleagues at the time was that they were not allowed to volunteer. This I believe has now changed. Certainly, working in a disaster zone is quite close to a war situation, and it would have been very useful to add to their experience, as well as providing useful staff.

I was in the last group of short-term volunteers, and most of the necessary acute surgery had been done when we arrived. There were still enormous problems of housing, feeding and continuing medical needs. This was made much worse by the outbreak of cholera some weeks later, which infected 665,000 people and killed a further 8,200 people. Reports now in 2020, ten years after the quake, are very depressing. Despite $10 billion donated from countries around the world there has apparently been minimal rebuilding, human and government depression is a very common problem, and there is increasing lawlessness within both the city and the country. The anaesthetist and I flew in and out via the Dominican Republic, which makes up about two-thirds of the island of Hispaniola. Because of the timing of the UN flights, we had a day in the capital, Santo Domingo, each way. On the way in we did not realise that the Dominican Republic, even without the damage from the earthquake, was in very much better condition than Haiti. On the way home this was very obvious. This was apparently due to the fact that in colonial days the Dominican Republic was a Spanish colony and had been far better treated before, on and after its independence than had Haiti, which had been French. The history of the area is fascinating as to possible reasons for the differences, even though the population is equivalent. The Dominican Republic now has a thriving tourism industry, Haiti, even before the quake, has none.

Those two days gave us a chance to visit Santo Domingo, and on our way home to go for a long walk to help in our recovery from the containment and horrors that we had seen in Haiti.

The Philippines Typhoon, 8 December 2013
After the Haiti earthquake, Professor Tony Redmond OBE had done a marvellous job with the British Government, extracting government funding for setting up and funding a national disaster relief team. This was known as the United Kingdom International Emergency Relief Team (UKIETR, later to become UK Med). The idea was that when the government needed a team to go to a disaster or war zone, then a fully trained and equipped team would be on instant readiness. Recruitment was open to any qualified health care professional for the training, but only experienced people would be sent overseas. I knew that there had always been a problem getting time off from the NHS, and with this new team there would be a number of people required on instant standby for two-week periods, and their locums in their hospitals would be found, and paid for, by the government. It was a marvellous idea, and it removed the need for the time and personnel that had been needed for fund-raising. Some of us had done the weekend training at the fire station training base at Chipping Norton organised by Tony Redmond and Dr Amy Hughes. And then came the Philippines typhoon.

Typhoon is an Asian word meaning 'Big Wind', and typhoons are known as hurricanes in the west. Every year each typhoon or hurricane is given a person's name, initially always female, but now of either sex.

Through the season the initial letter of the name moves through the alphabet.

The Philippines regularly have typhoons, but Typhoon Haijan in December 2013 was the strongest ever recorded there, with a steady wind speed of 195mph and gusting at greater than 235mph. The wind itself caused very severe damage, but the 6,240 deaths were mainly caused by the 13ft-high storm surge that entered the harbour at Tacloban on Leyte Island.

The British team consisted of three surgeons, two anaesthetists, four accident and emergency doctors and four nurses, and was mobilised a few days later. We met at Heathrow and were given our emergency tents, sleeping bags, etc. I also took my basic skin grafting equipment. We flew out to Manila and then to Cebu, a city to which I had previously been as visiting professor. There the team split into two. Half were to go to Tacloban to assess and treat those injured by the storm surge, and the other half, including the three A&E doctors and me, were to join the British destroyer HMS *Daring* to visit various islands to assess the numbers of deaths and injuries and the requirements for treatment in the many islands which had been completely cut off. At the same time emergency humanitarian packs of food and necessities were to be distributed by the Navy.

HMS *Daring* (*see* Plate 6.9) was the first of the Type 45 air defence destroyers and was launched in 2006. At the time of the typhoon, it was returning from Australia, where it had joined in the celebrations of the centenary of their Navy, and was diverted to aid in the Philippines. We boarded her at the port in rigid inflatable boats (RIBs). Unfortunately, on our way out a serious injury occurred to the leader of our team, Professor Tony Redmond. He was not used to riding in a RIB in rough seas, and sat down instead of standing, and a heavy jolt caused him to have a spinal fracture. In great pain he continued to lead the team but it took him many months to recover. As we approached the ship, it grew remarkably larger. We were offered a lift up in a bosun's chair, but instead we all climbed a moving rope ladder without falling into the sea. We met the captain and his crew and were assigned a bunk and introduced to the wardroom. As was to happen every night for the rest of the week, we sailed to the next affected islands, where we arrived the next morning.

More than a hundred islands had been affected by the storm. For each one the plan was to move a team ashore, either by RIB if there was a suitable landing area, or by the ship's Lynx helicopter. Once onshore,

Dr Amy Hughes made contact with the Headman to assess the number of people who had died or needed help. She then asked permission to set up an out-patient clinic, normally in the local school if it was still standing. The other two doctors, the nurses and I then got on with treating patients. Whilst all this was happening, the Navy, often with the goods slung below the helicopter, brought in the humanitarian packs which were then distributed. I understood later that in Tacloban there had been riots when the packs arrived, and the disorder was very difficult to control. The islanders who received their packs from us caused no problems at all. And I do not think that it was the sight of military uniforms that had that effect. The navy personnel were often to be found repairing buildings, and particularly schools, a task which they very much enjoyed (*see* Plate 6.10). Several said to me that it made a marvellous change from their normal work, and that they felt privileged to be able to help. The summary of our findings, which was remarkably constant across the islands we visited, was that very few people had died, and the deaths were more often caused by heart attacks than by building collapse or wind damage. There were some fractures and lacerations, most of which had been treated already. We did some re-dressings and opened infected wounds, and then for the remainder of the clinic saw patients with a variety of longstanding medical and surgical conditions. Many of these took me back forty years to my time in Africa. Unfortunately we did not have the relevant drugs or equipment to treat all of them.

In the Philippines cold is never a problem, since cooking can be done over fires fuelled by wood, of which there was then a vast new surplus. The main problems were obtaining clean drinking water, since most sources had been polluted, and the damage to the fishing boats. Both of these were serious. Polluted drinking water can cause severe medical problems, and as fishing was the islanders' major source of both protein and income, the fact that on many islands most of their boats had been destroyed or severely damaged would be a problem for months or years to come. Many houses were also damaged and electricity supplies cut off.

Our work was simple, safe and not particularly stressful. When we returned to base we met the Tacloban team. Life had been very different for them. They had been living in their tents, and food was a variable occurrence. There were large numbers of injured patients, several of whom needed surgery. Afterwards it was clear that my skills as a plastic surgeon would have been more useful there, as some of the patients would have had a greater benefit. I have expanded on this in my summary.

Overall, it was an interesting and useful visit. It also gave credence to the British Government for the formation and funding of the idea of the relief team. It is possible that this was the first time when civilian and military teams worked closely together and was without doubt to the benefit of the patients. I sincerely hope that it will become normal practice in the future. We were one of several countries which sent teams, and the coordination for this disaster was, I thought, better than that in Haiti.

In summary, 6,240 people died in the disaster and more than 23,000 were injured. More than 6 million people were displaced or needed their homes rebuilt as more than a million homes had been damaged or destroyed.

We returned home in time for Christmas, and a period of reflection.

South Sudan Tanker Explosion, 17 September 2015

About two days after this disaster occurred I received a call from Professor Tony Redmond asking if I could be available to fly to Juba, the capital of South Sudan, to assess the direct consequences of a fuel tanker explosion that had happened near the town of Maridi, close to the southern border between South Sudan and Uganda. I said that I would be happy to go, and asked for any further information as I had seen nothing about it on the British television news.

What had happened was that a petrol tanker had crashed, and the local villagers had moved in to steal the fuel. There had been an explosion when the fuel ignited. At least 206 people had died, and some 280 people had been injured, nearly all of whom had burns. There was later an unconfirmed report that the explosion might have been caused by a policeman firing his gun into the air in an attempt to control the crowd, and the flash ignited the fumes.

South Sudan was the newest country in the world. It became independent in 2011, when a long-standing civil war caused by both tribal and religious differences with Sudan was settled. The new country had been divided into ten districts and held sixty tribes. There were still major disagreements happening, and there was an attempt to reduce the ten districts to four. The accident happened near Maridi, 151 miles to the west of Juba. The more seriously injured patients were taken to the local hospital, where a team from Médecins sans Frontières (MSF) was looking after them. Unfortunately when the MSF team arrived, it found that the hospital had been completely stripped of equipment and staff during a local tribal war, all of which had to be imported by MSF.

Medical Care in Disasters and Wars

Although only a small percentage of the injured were children, it had been agreed that Save the Children (SAVE) would organise the British response, presumably because it had a long-standing and large presence in Juba. After a meeting in London, I flew out via Dubai and Addis Ababa to Juba with two SAVE staff, with the request to assess the number of injured and how many would require further surgery, and what would be the staff and equipment requirements needed for this.

The SAVE team was based in a large building close to the hotel in which we were staying. I met the local team who had been there for many months, had an official 'safeguarding' SAVE tutorial – to complement my UN, St John Ambulance and Scout ones, which not surprisingly were all very repetitive – and then we were driven to the Government Hospital where we met a local doctor, and then visited the burned patients on three wards (two adult and one children's ward). There were about sixty adults and six children. It must be said that medical and nursing personnel in many less developed countries are used to treating burns, which are very common injuries. The patients were being managed by exposure of the burned areas. This is rarely used in Britain, but is very common in many parts of the world. The main disadvantages are that it is more painful, particularly in the early stages, and slightly more likely to cause infection. The advantages are that it is much less expensive and needs less nursing time for dressings. The majority of the patients in the Juba Hospital were partial thickness burns and were about halfway through the healing process. There was one child with very severe deep burns of one arm and hand, and three adults who would require skin grafting. One of the three was severely burned, with a risk of dying from his injuries. There were no cases of inhalation burns, which as the incident had been outside was not unusual. The nursing care was clearly good, but as is so often the case in developing countries there was a severe shortage of anaesthetists. The only one there was somewhat elderly, and had retired on ill-health grounds two years previously. There was also a shortage of surgeons, as the senior members of the Ministry of Health and the senior surgeons were all visiting Maridi at the time. I had met the senior general surgeon when he had been on an exchange to St Mary's Hospital on the Isle of Wight, arranged by an old colleague of mine, Mr Tim Walsh, and it would have been useful to have discussed the problems with him. There was a very helpful doctor employed by the UN, and it was through her that plans were made. Apart from very minor tidy-ups on the burned child's arm and re-dressings, I had little clinical work to do.

On the assessment of the equipment there was a lack of skin grafting tools. SAVE had sent out a large load of general surgery tools which were not relevant for this disaster, but no doubt were well received.

Whilst there I had to be registered as a medical practitioner. This took nearly two days and three pages of my passport. I have operated in many countries of the world with no local registration, but at least South Sudan had got this organised, but it did use the time and effort of one fully qualified doctor – not perhaps the best use of a short resource. After writing my report, and knowing that an American plastic surgeon and an anaesthetist were to follow me for the necessary surgery, I flew home.

Two things happened later. I saw a report from MSF, and the total number of dead was 206 and there were 280 injured, of whom 125 needed admission. After my return, with a trainee plastic surgeon, Mr O. Sawyer, we wrote a paper on tanker injuries, which was published in the journal *Burns*. In the previous fifteen years there had been twenty-five incidents in seventeen countries reported in the general and medical press. With the exception of a small incident in Australia, these were all in developing countries. The worst had been in the Congo, when 220 people died, and the South Sudan incident was the next most severe. In all of these incidents a total of 1,415 people had died, but only 851 injuries were reported. However, eleven of the incident reports only reported deaths. This is another example of a common reporting problem making analysis and recommendations difficult.

Recommendations for Disaster Management

After each of the disasters in which I was involved there was a form of feedback, either as a meeting or as a written report. These would record what had gone well and what problems had occurred. Suggestions were then made to try to prevent the same problems in the future.

Using the experience from the six disasters in which I had been involved, the following are the recommendations that I would make.

Disaster Planning

Firstly there needs to be a plan to respond to any local emergency, and secondly there needs to be a plan to give aid away from the base, either in other parts of the country or overseas. In many parts of the world all the main hospitals, all the cities or counties and all the countries have a disaster plan in place. These are frequently less than perfect. For example, from the literature it is known that at least 50 per cent of disasters with

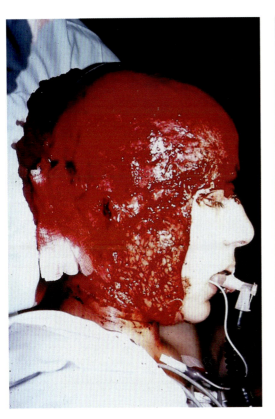
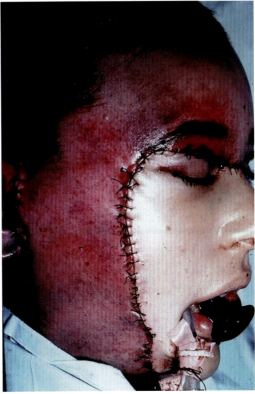
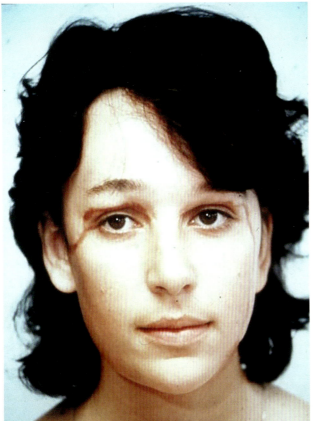

Plate 1.1. The original problem: major loss of scalp.

Plate 1.2. After replantation, and ...

Plate 1.3. ... Six months later.

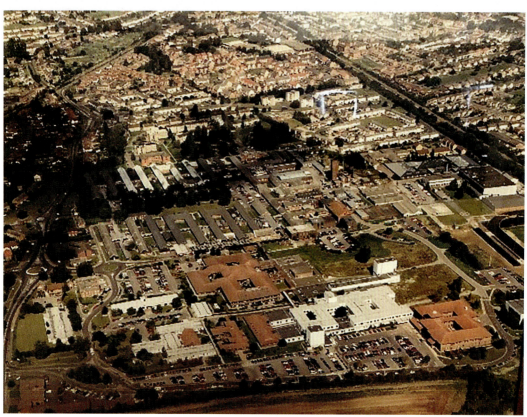

Plate 2.1. Stoke Mandeville Hospital in the 1990s. The old huts are in the centre, with the new Spinal Unit in the centre foreground. The new hospital is in the foreground on the right.

Plate 2.2. The large surgical team required for a major burn operation.

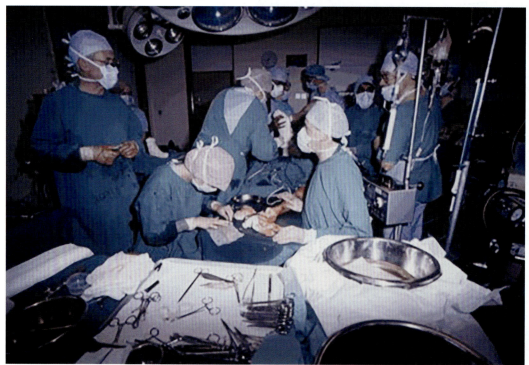

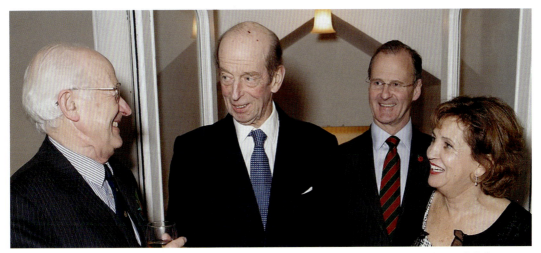

Plate 3.1. Professor Anthony Roberts (President), HRH the Duke of Kent (Patron), Lord Calum Graham (Chairman) and Lady Graham.

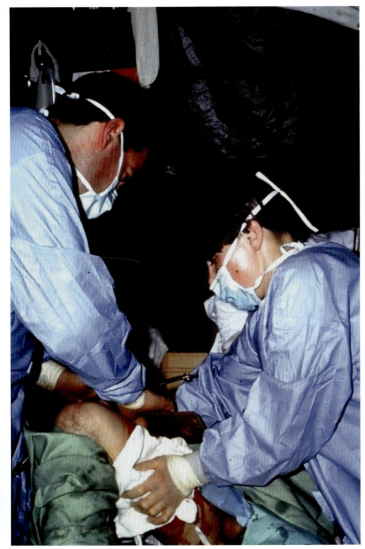

Plate 5.1. Squadron Leader Scerri and his assistant operating in Saudi Arabia.

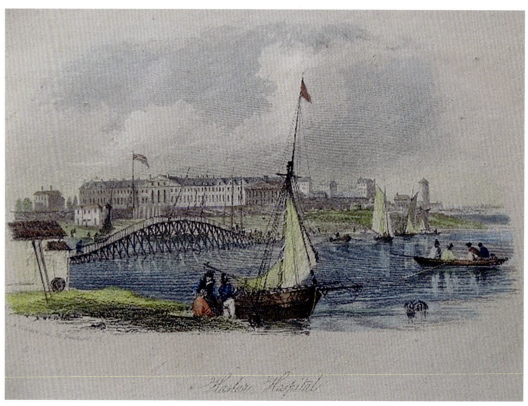

Plate 5.2. An early print showing the Royal Hospital, Haslar.

Plate 5.3. The Royal Hospital, Haslar's celebration of 250 years. (*By courtesy of the artist, Colin M. Baxter Esq.*)

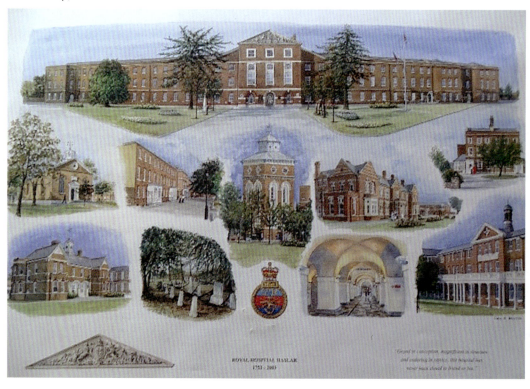

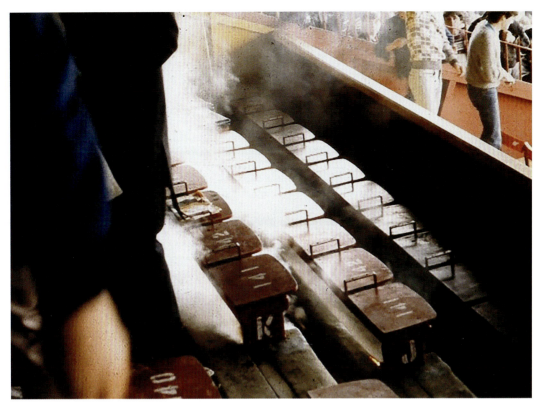

Plate 6.1. The start of the Bradford fire. It was probably caused by a discarded cigarette end.

Plate 6.2. About four minutes later.

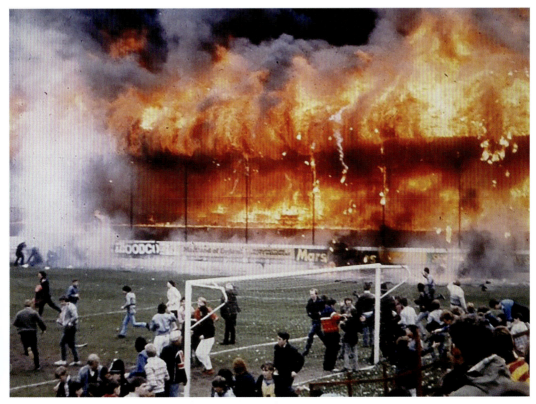

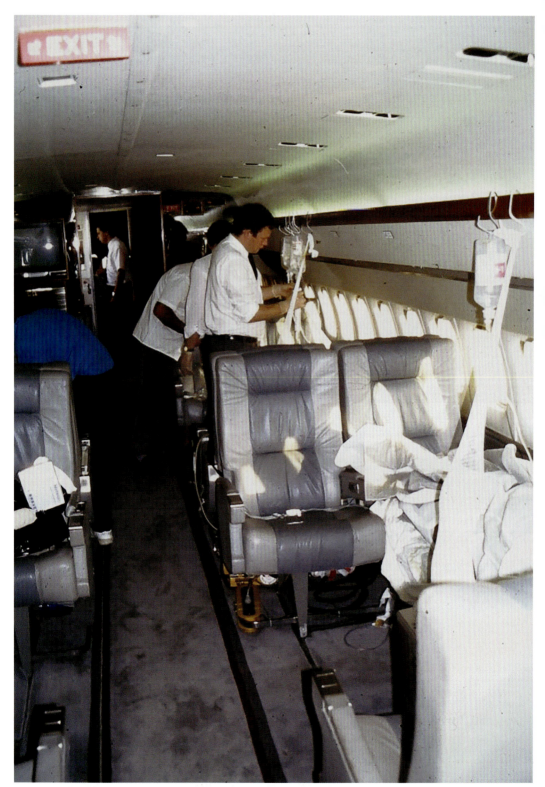
Plate 6.3. A commercial airliner modified for burn patient transfer.

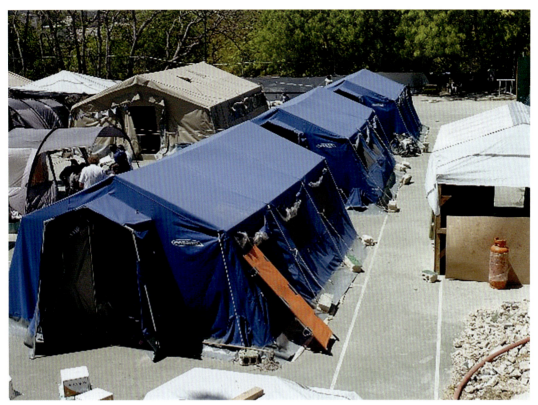

Plate 6.4. The Wimbledon Hospital in Haiti.

Plate 6.5. An orthopaedic surgeon with a happy healing patient.

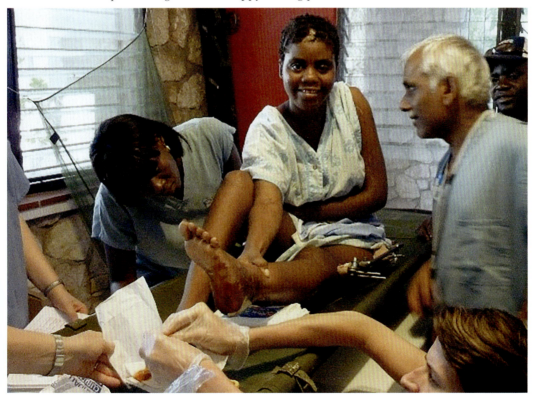

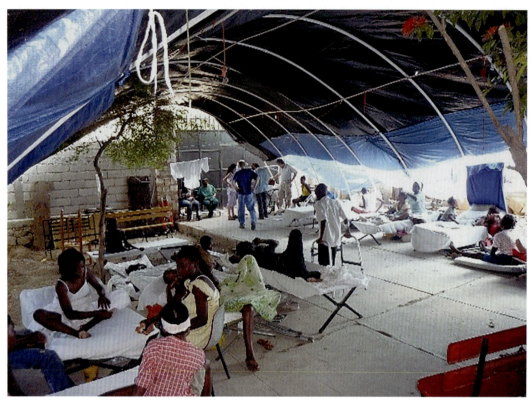

Plate 6.6. The Heartline American Hospital.

Plate 6.7. ShelterBox supplies.

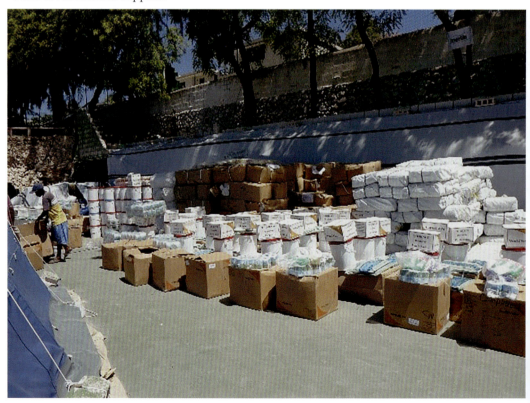

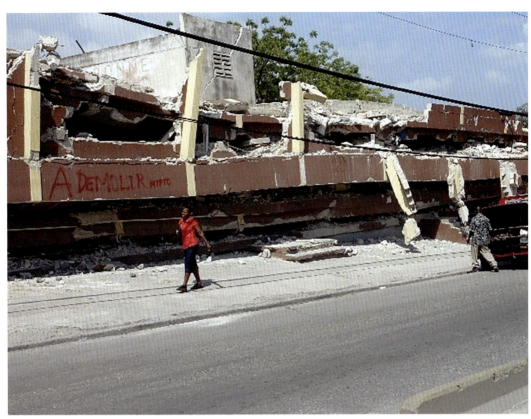

Plate 6.8. The remains of a five-storey building.

Plate 6.9. HMS *Daring* and the helicopter.

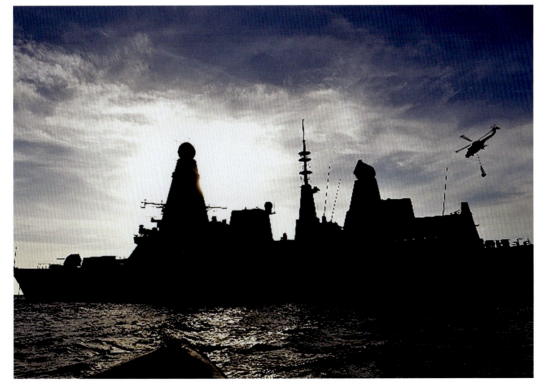

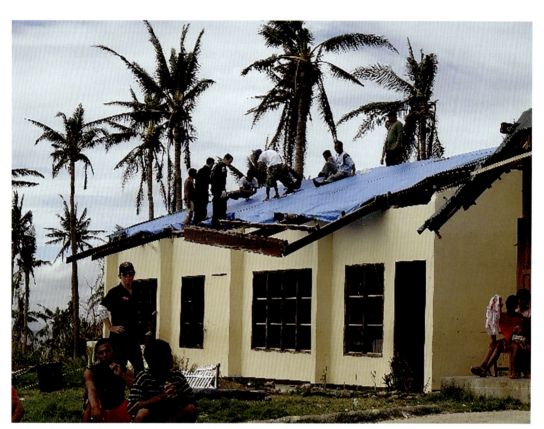

Plate 6.10. Naval personnel repairing the local school roof.

Plate 6.11. Illegal 'Maybe Airlines' passport stamp.

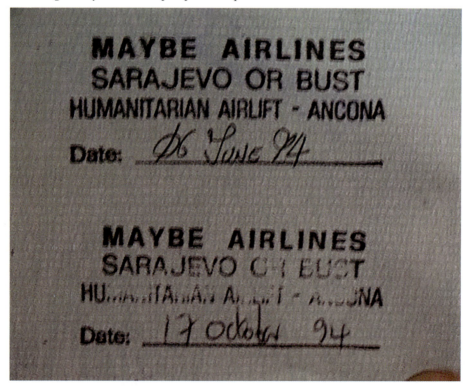

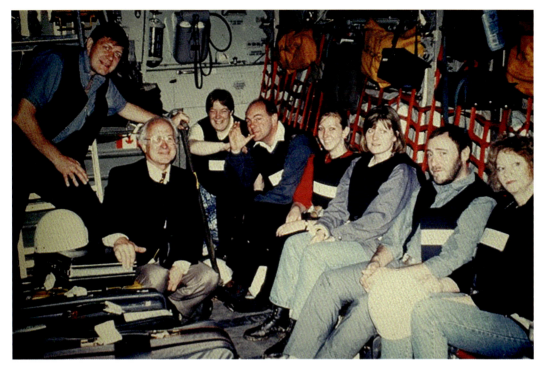

Plate 6.12. The team in the RAF Hercules.

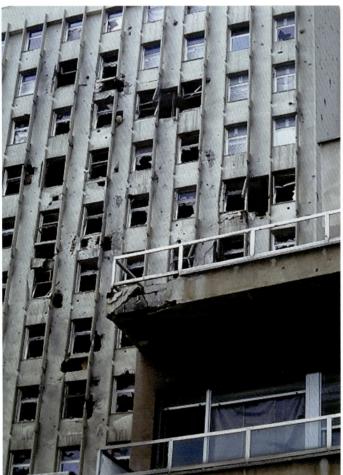

Plate 6.13. The 'Swiss Cheese Hospital'.

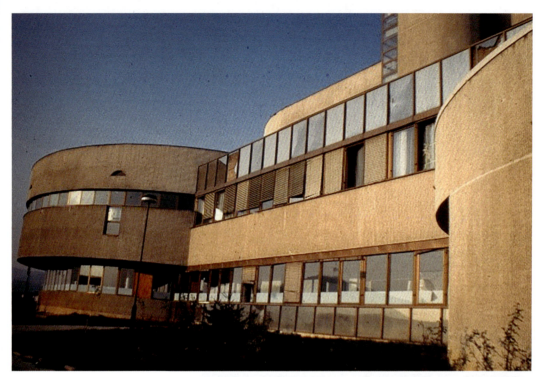

Plate 6.14. The University of Sarajevo Hospital.

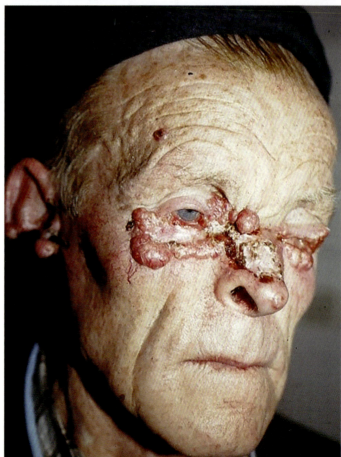

Plate 6.15. Skin cancers. These would have been easily curable years earlier.

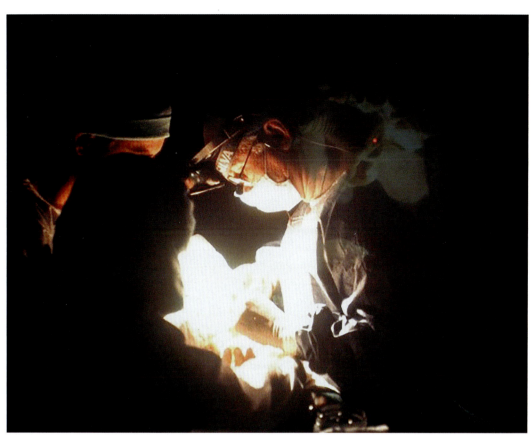

Plate 6.16. Operating by torchlight: a new experience for me.

Plate 6.17. The Olympic ice-stadium that served as the United Nations base.

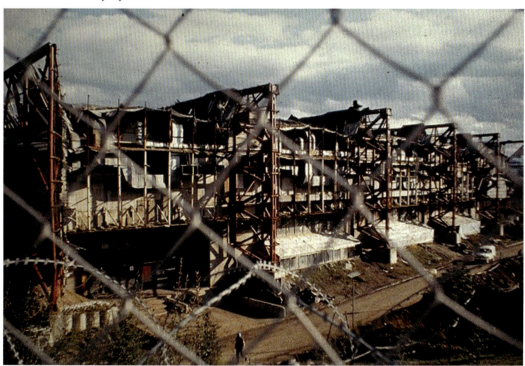

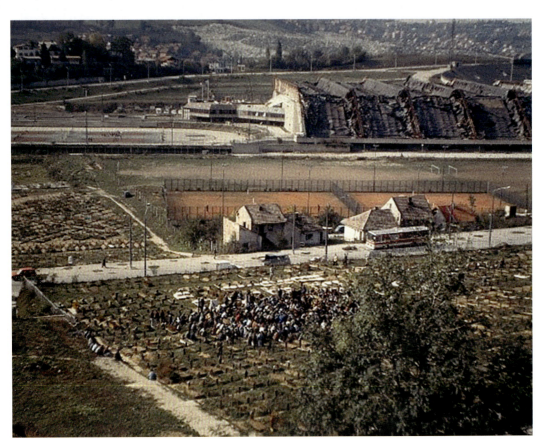

Plate 6.18. The main Sarajevo graveyard during the war.

Plate 6.19. The Old City with the Serb lines above.

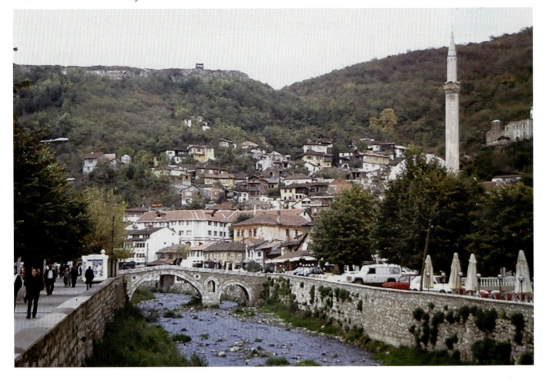

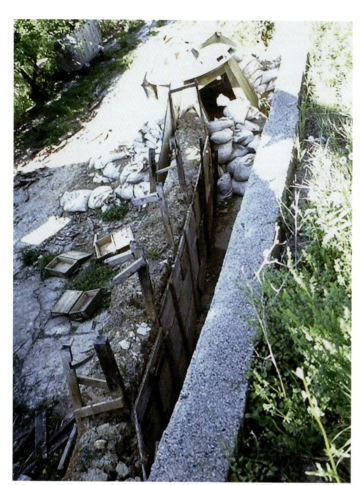

Plate 6.20. The old Serb trenches above Sarajevo.

Plate 6.21. The graveyard after the war, with stone replacing wood.

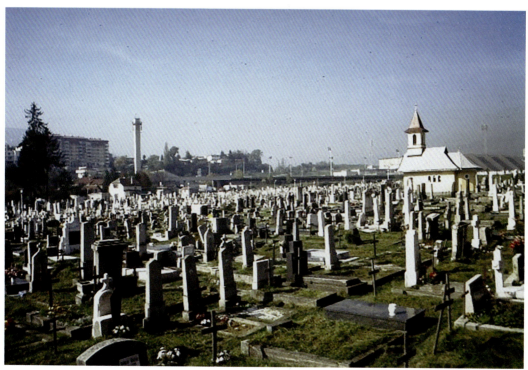

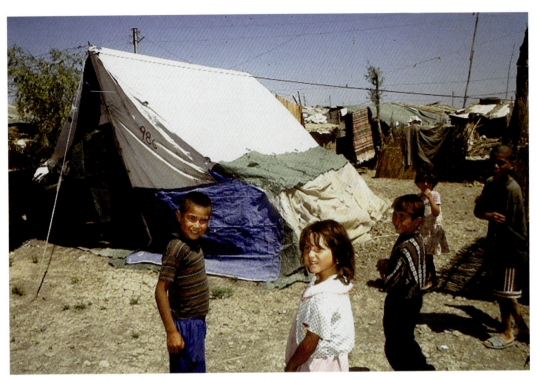

Plate 6.22. A small area in a large tented camp, Azerbaijan.

Plate 8.1. St John First Aid Post in 1940.

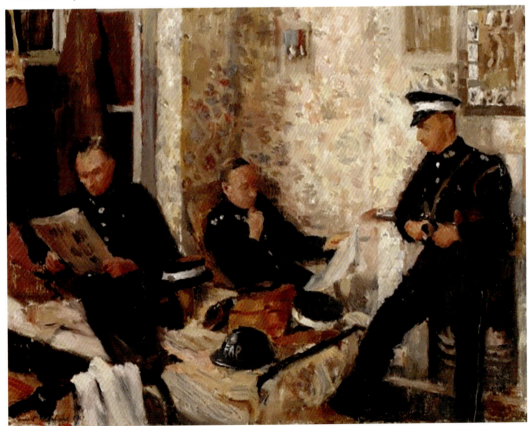

surviving patients involve burn injuries, yet many plans do not include a burn expert to do the original triage (sorting of patients). Triage by inexperienced people can mean that patients with no chance of survival can be put into intensive care beds that would more appropriately be used for those patients who could survive. A useful division between out-and in-patients in terms of burns is 5 per cent, which will cover most situations as long as there are no inhalation problems or other injuries. I would add from personal experience that triage can be very difficult. The essential task is to assess all the casualties so that appropriate help can be called. It is, though, extremely difficult not to treat the first person who needs immediate care. Disaster plans should also be practised at least biannually, and particularly at staff change times of year. I had seen this done superbly at Hadassah Hospital in Jerusalem (*see* Chapter 9).

Communications.
In the Bradford disaster the problem of communication was highlighted. Since then much has changed with the introduction of long-range bleeps and mobile phones, both in the United Kingdom and around the world. These are not completely reliable even in cities. It is not possible to stress the importance of communication in disaster or war situations. One solution to this is satellite phones, which have been used successfully and should be part of the standard equipment of all aid teams.

Nurses
The initial thinking when a disaster happens is that the major requirements are beds, surgeons, physicians and anaesthetists. But nurses are also essential, both at the beginning and, more importantly, later on when dressings need to be replaced. This is particularly important with burn casualties.

Relief Teams
There is an enormous willingness to help from countries around the world when major disasters occur. But here experience, equipment and training will all make the help of greater value. The strongest advice that I would give is that nobody who is not a consultant in a British hospital or the equivalent around the world should be part of a team. Their value is enhanced by their years of experience, particularly if they have worked in developing countries or overseas where the most modern equipment may not be available. The presence of a plastic surgeon with burn and reconstructive experience will always be of advantage to a team as skin damage

Plastic Surgery in Wars, Disasters and Civilian Life

is a common problem in trauma situations. In developed countries a plastic surgeon will often plan a series of operations on a patient. In disaster areas there is usually only the opportunity for one operation, and again experience can enable them to do as much as is usefully possible in that one operation. During the recent war in Afghanistan a plastic surgeon was added to the team in the British military hospital, and he operated in theatre more often than either the general or the orthopaedic surgeon.

Logistics
Only with experience have I realised the importance of several things. The first is language, where effective translation, ideally using a locally recruited person who can help with the social problems that will occur, is vital. Secondly, a good logistician is crucial to ensure that the necessary equipment is as available as possible, and this may include a tented hospital and arrangements for transport, sleeping and feeding staff.

Funding
When government funding is available, then a major pressure is removed from the organisers. When charities are involved, they obviously need to raise money, but I believe this should be done in the home country, rather than through charity workers present at the scene of the disaster, which may preclude additional clinical people being present.

The Roman poet Ovid's comments about the press are given at the end of the chapter, and totally reinforce my own experience.

Wars

Medical care during wars is often very different from that following natural or man-made disasters. Certainly for the attacking country or group there is sufficient time to plan for the onset of the attack, although this also applies in most cases to the country or group being attacked. The planning involved can be complex, particularly if the areas in which the attacks are occurring are some distance from major cities, or lack good ground or air communications. The other problem that is now fully recognised is that until recently (after the Second World War), medical care of the troops was more necessary for normal illnesses and accidents as these were the causes of more deaths than war injuries.

Medical care in wars has at least four stages. Firstly, injured personnel have to be removed from the front line, having been given basic first aid. The second stage is a base hospital, which may already have been in existence or is set up specifically for the attack. The third stage is that the more severely injured or ill personnel can be removed to a major hospital some distance from the attack zone or transferred away, often now by air, to a hospital where major care is possible. The fourth stage of care following war injuries can be rehabilitation in specialist centres. For many years rehabilitation in Britain took place at Headley Court in Surrey. The military forces of many countries have these lines of evacuation and treatment set up, and their use is frequently practised. All military medical systems regularly analyse, from their own experience and that of others, the changing patterns in military medical care caused by the development and use of new weapons.

This pattern of medical care can obviously be upset if the attacking troops are either rebuffed or have been so successful that they have advanced more rapidly than the evacuation lines can be developed. This is, however, much more likely to be a problem for the country or group that is being attacked, and particularly if they are being defeated. Furthermore, the established set-up of medical care in a whole country or region can be partially or even completely disrupted by the effects of warfare, and this can include psychological problems which may be caused by the fighting.

Medical care in war has been well studied and is widely published in the literature.

During my career as a consultant surgeon I was involved in four wars. These had a profound effect both on me and often on the people with whom I was working.

The First Gulf War, 1990–1991
The First Gulf War between the United States and its allies and Iraq was fought in 1990 and 1991. My report on my involvement with this war is given in Chapter 5.

The Bosnian War, 1992–1995
My visits to Sarajevo were some of the greatest events of my life. How they came about is interesting. Professor Tony Redmond from UK Med visited Sarajevo at the beginning of the ceasefire period towards the end of the Bosnian War in early 1994. After discussion, there was an opinion that there were three things for which help was most needed. One of these was plastic and reconstructive surgery. The call therefore went out from the British Association of Plastic Surgeons for people willing to volunteer to go and help. I volunteered, and was then asked to recruit a team of people to go with me. I therefore asked around my colleagues and to my amazement and gratitude everybody that I asked immediately volunteered. The

team that I took mostly consisted of colleagues from Stoke Mandeville, with whom I had worked for many years. They were Dr Richard Bunsell (consultant anaesthetist), Sister Jacky Benson (theatre sister), Maria Clarke (occupational therapist and splint expert), Michael Hunt (senior operating department assistant from the Chiltern Hospital), Brenner Hay (a resuscitation officer) and two physiotherapists, Jan and another one from a different unit who had been added to my team. Richard had a very new baby and Maria had no travel experience, but their volunteering was instantaneous. It turned out that we were also to have a television crew with us from BBC 4. After obtaining passports where required and having the appropriate vaccinations, we worked out what we needed in the way of equipment and arranged to travel from Aylesbury to London Heathrow in June 1994, where we met Professor Redmond and the television crew. There we collected the equipment that we might need and set off firstly to Rome and then to Ancona, where we spent the night in an excellent hotel. We had one interesting experience in Rome whilst we were changing planes. By this stage we were equipped with flak jackets and flak helmets in United Nations blue. As we went through the airport screening in Rome, three people went through in full flak equipment before one of the staff there asked, 'Where are you going?' We replied, 'Sarajevo,' and they said, 'Okay; no problems.'

In the hotel we got to know the television crew, consisting of the director Jeremy Llewellyn Jones, his assistant Emma and the cameraman John. After an excellent dinner, the very experienced television cameraman started filling his pockets with everything that was left on the table. We said, 'Have you not had enough?' to which his reply was, 'I don't know where my next meal is coming from – do you?' And so we all filled up our pockets with whatever was lying around. John, who had spent many years working in war zones and disaster areas, was actually living in Belfast, where he had met his wife on one of his many visits. He was a very experienced man indeed and the ideal person to give us confidence.

The next day we went to Ancona airport, where we were briefed by the Royal Air Force as we were due to fly to Sarajevo in a C130 Hercules. The Royal Air Force, which was backed by the Royal Canadian Air Force, was known as Maybe Airlines: it may be flying – or maybe not. Our passports were stamped with the Maybe Airlines stamp, which was totally illegal, but I'm delighted to say they continue to do so (see Plate 6.11). The other thing that I remember at the airport was a hand-written notice entitled 'Ten good reasons for visiting Sarajevo.' Unfortunately I did not take a photograph of this but I still remember some of the good reasons, which included,

- There are no fat ladies in Sarajevo
- There are no speed limits in Sarajevo
- It is a good place to diet

Unfortunately I cannot remember the remainder, but it did cheer us all up on our way out to a great unknown. As well as our personal gear, we were taking some medical equipment and useful apparatus such as computers, copying machines, etc. The RCAF Hercules had seats along each side, and a large load of cargo in the middle. The cargo had been brought in through the back door, which hinged down. And so, sitting in our flak jackets and helmets, we took off in the extremely noisy aeroplane towards Sarajevo (*see* Plate 6.12). Unfortunately the Hercules went wrong on the way over, and they could not turn the excess heating off that was gently cooking us. We therefore returned to Ancona. After a delay of a couple of hours we transferred to a Royal Air Force Hercules and flew back towards Sarajevo. Any of us who wanted were invited into the cockpit and had a guided tour of the cockpit and some lovely views over the clouds. Apparently there were two ways of approaching Sarajevo, as it necessitated flying over Serb-held territory; this could be dangerous as they might take pot-shots at any incoming plane. Either one came in at a very high altitude and dived down at a very steep angle, pulling up at the last moment to land on the runway, or one came in at a very low altitude, as we did, because of low cloud (almost fog). Just before landing, as the plane emerged out of the fog, I did notice that rockets were fired from both wingtips when we were about 100ft above the ground.

When I asked about the rockets, I discovered that this was to decoy any heatseeking missiles fired at us by the Serbs. We stopped after landing without mishap, and then to my amazement the Hercules began reversing its propellers and was able to back up. We therefore reversed rapidly into an area that was safe from fire from any Serbian ground forces as it was behind a wall of sandbags. The gear was taken off the plane and we followed. It was an interesting flight – at least the aircrew had done it before!

Two Land Rovers were packed with our personal gear and the computers, printers and medical equipment. We then set off to drive the 4 miles to the city centre, seeing severely damaged houses on both sides of the road. Unfortunately, after about half a mile we were stopped by some

Serbian troops. On the opposite side of the road were Italian peacekeeping troops, who had been given the ridiculous order that they were not to shoot at anybody unless they were first shot at. The Serbs therefore robbed us of all the equipment we were taking in for our work, but actually left us our own personal gear, perhaps thinking that they were being kind! This was the first time that we had rifles pointed at us to make certain that we did as commanded by the Serbian troops. And this was supposed to be a country under ceasefire.

We were then driven to our accommodation – a combination of the Holiday Inn and a rented apartment closer to the centre of the city. The Holiday Inn was a large yellow building. It had excellent air-conditioning from previous gunfire over the past few years. At this time in the cease-fire the international press had moved in in a large way, and in fact our BBC team stayed there for the whole of the two weeks. Some of our team joined me in an apartment on the first night, and the rest joined us the following day. The TV crew met many of their colleagues from around the world, including Kate Adie, whom I had met after the Bradford Football Club fire.

The drive from the airport to Sarajevo city had been very depressing with the damage to the buildings, but in the city centre the damage was very much greater, with almost no glass left in any windows. From the Holiday Inn one could see the hill just the other side of the river where the Serbs were very close and looking down on the city. I did not appreciate how close they were until after the war had finished and I went up into their trenches to collect some shell cases as souvenirs. These mementos I still have. They were only about 300–400 yards away. Like all troops, they were likely to get drunk, and fire indiscriminately at any windows which they could see that were still intact. The United Nations had provided plastic to cover virtually all of the windows in the city. That night we all had dinner in the Holiday Inn, of a very reasonable standard, and then went to bed wondering what was going to happen the following day.

There were two main hospitals in Sarajevo. The military hospital in the centre of town had become known as the Swiss Cheese Hospital (*see* Plate 6.13), and one can see why from the photograph as it was the shape of a lump of cheese with a large number of holes in it. It turned out that only the basement and a small part of the third floor facing away from the Serb lines were of any use. Working there was a quite remarkable general surgeon, Dr Mohammed, who had worked there day and night for the past four years and was extremely accomplished. There had also been two military plastic surgeons working there, but no longer. The other hospital was the University hospital (*see* Plate 6.14) up the hill from the centre of town, and apparently this had been intentionally left almost undamaged by the Serbs so that they could take it over as a working hospital when they conquered the city. Before the war Sarajevo had been an excellent medical centre. In the field of plastic surgery alone there were twelve consultants in the university which was greater than the number in any unit in Britain at that time. It turned out that all of these had gone, either because they were Serbs, or because they were Bosnians who had been killed or injured. The department there was therefore run by a dentist, Dr Hujic, with five or six junior trainee surgeons assisting.

The following morning our team turned up at the Swiss Cheese Hospital and were met by Dr Nakas, the Director (and the brother of Dr Mohammed). It was not a particularly warm welcome, but we were shown round the small amount of the hospital that remained functional and then introduced to two Austrian surgeons from the major trauma hospital in Vienna. Both they and we got the impression that the locals did not really know what to do with us, as the only surgery occurring in the hospital was general surgery. Professor Redmond therefore went off to the University Hospital to see if he could find a role for us to play there, and I started operating with the Austrians on a severe hand injury. It was very successful, and this changed the whole atmosphere. It turned out later that another European country, which should perhaps remain nameless, two weeks earlier had sent over a team of, in effect, surgical trainees and they had left several disasters behind. This really verified the rule in England that no trainee goes on missions such as this, and ideally no consultant with less than five years' experience at that level. As one of the local juniors put it to me later when we had become friends, 'Do surgeons from X [not to be mentioned] only operate on Africans – because all their flaps were black?' This is never good news – in fact, it's an absolute surgical disaster as it meant that the operation had not only failed but also made the situation worse.

The other patient that I remember from the Swiss Cheese Hospital was an example of what frequently happens in war and disaster situations, when 'ordinary' problems are either ignored or given lower priority. This is now happening in 2020 in the UK and in many other parts of the world as the Covid-19 pandemic is taking over. A typical example can be seen in Plate 6.15, which shows severe and multiple facial skin cancers. These would have been easy to treat in the early stages, but not three or four years down the line. Another patient was brought in by an orthopaedic surgeon with a large deep swelling on the front of his wrist, which had affected his sensation and thumb movement. The surgeon thought that this was a cancer within the nerve and was going to remove the whole lump, leaving the patient with little sensation and reduced movement in the hand. I had seen and treated similar lumps in nerves in England and knew that the chances were that it was benign and non-malignant. With one of Richard Bunsell's arm blocks and a tourniquet, I dissected out the lump from within the nerve and we took it back to England to confirm that it was a benign Schwannoma. Leaving the rest of the nerve behind gave the patient an excellent chance of a full recovery and I received the thanks of both patient and surgeon, and our status improved further.

Towards the end of the first week Tony Redmond had done his excellent publicity work at the University Hospital, and I suspect there was also some communication between the hospitals. I therefore went up the hill with our team and the BBC crew to do a clinic to select patients for surgery the following week. My original brief was that I was going to reconstruct patients with contractures after burn injuries. In fact there were no such patients in the clinic as almost no patients with major burns had survived. Dealing with such burns when they occur requires both knowledge and the availability of appropriate treatment and equipment, which in the war situation had simply not been available. Most of the patients in the clinic had been injured some months or years previously and had suffered severe damage to a nerve or nerves and often bones in an arm or arms. This type of late damage I rarely saw in England and it required a very different type of surgery where tendons are redeployed to enable them to have a different function on the wrist or fingers. I had luckily taken an appropriate textbook with me and worked out what would be the best operation for several of the patients. In my six weeks of operating in Sarajevo I did more tendon transfers than in the rest of my career.

It became apparent during this time that although basic equipment was either missing or needed to be cleaned and reused, the staff maintained excellent sterility and the trainee surgeons were keen and two or three were excellent. Interestingly, with one exception the anaesthetists were all ladies and all good. When we got to know them socially, and the ice had melted somewhat, in discussion they said that surgery was considered a male prerogative and the females became anaesthetists. Anaesthesia was an interesting problem. When Richard Bunsell, our anaesthetist, saw the apparatus, which had not been serviced for four years, and noted the lack of availability of oxygen he went somewhat pale. But being Richard, he got on with the help of the local anaesthetists, particularly Dr Zjelka Knesevic, who took us under her very capable wing and who spoke flawless English. Richard was particularly useful in that he was able to teach them brachial block anaesthesia, of which they had very little experience. This method uses a local anaesthetic to put an arm to sleep; it does not require oxygen, and was therefore much safer. There were other problems in the hospital. All of the staff were unpaid. People worked because they were needed, and the only advantage was that food was provided. They smoked to reduce hunger pains. Washing hands before operating was made difficult when the water supply was cut off, and operating was made even more difficult when the electricity supply ceased. The local doctors were used to this and simply put a large torch on my head (*see* Plate 6.16). With my African experience, these limitations were less of a problem for me than they would have been for most visiting surgeons. We also had to get used to the explosions that were still happening all around the hospital; these could be somewhat distracting when embarking on a delicate part of the operation. It surprised me how quickly we learned to ignore these distractions.

Working with the BBC TV crew was interesting. I had done some television work before, but only speaking and being interviewed. Having the cameraman in theatre was a new twist. Luckily John was very experienced and in no way affected my surgery. We had already agreed, jokingly, that if he did not get his filming right first time, I was not going to do a re-run of the operation for him. The result became the first edition of a five edition programme called 'Siege Doctors' on BBC4.

On the wards the nursing was superb. The senior sister became a good friend (as I have said before, it is always an excellent idea for a doctor to make friends with the ward sister) and spoke excellent English, as did all the doctors and most of the nurses. Sister told me that what had upset her the most was that a shell had hit her apartment and wrecked her wardrobe, ruining all her clothes hanging within. She still turned out immaculately, as was amazingly normal for the ladies in a city with virtually no outside links and certainly no functioning shops. There was just one link – a tunnel under the Serb lines near the airport, through which food and essential supplies were brought. One of the junior trainee surgeons with whom I was working offered me a trip through the tunnel. Unfortunately I mentioned the offer to Robert Barnett, the British Ambassador at the time, and he asked me not to go as it could have caused the UN some embarrassment as all those using the tunnel were being filmed by the Serbs. I now much regret the missed opportunity. In 2020 the tunnel is now a tourist attraction.

The Ambassador, who was from my old college St Catharine's in Cambridge, had an excellent local young lady as his translator and assistant. He told me that her way of relieving her stress was to dress as a peasant and then go walkabout for a few days in the countryside behind the Serb lines. Very luckily she was not caught. After the war she married one of the best local trainee plastic surgeons and they emigrated to Norway, where he is now working as a consultant plastic surgeon.

Our team would have been happy to operate 12 or more hours a day, but the local doctors and nurses who had been working seven days a week continuously for four years were happier with 8-hour operating days. This gave us some time for socialising. Once a week the British Ambassador and his team provided a dinner, which was well supplied with excellent wine. Some of this was brought in from Serbia by the International Red Cross doctor. During one of these dinners the fuel from our Land Rover was siphoned out whilst we were dining. However, the major part of our social life was organised by the anaesthetists, particularly Zjelka, and by Mrs Nadja Kurtagic, who was our contact with the Bosnian Ministry of Health. I was still in contact with her until her death a few months ago, and remain in touch with her daughter, who now lives in London. It was possible to walk around some parts of the city during the day when the Serb lines were far enough away, or at night as there were no street lights. And it was a beautiful city – or had been before the shelling and fires which were the only way of disposing of rubbish. The city was in three parts, the ancient Ottoman Empire part, the Austro-Hungarian Empire part and a much less attractive modern part where the architecture was Russian-influenced. It was possible to buy goods from local people, such as jewellery or in my case two paintings. The prices were embarrassingly low as the money, dollars, was urgently needed. For the only time in my life I did not bargain. Parts of the city were definitely out of bounds in the daytime. Sniper's Alley was appropriately named and definitely not recommended. It could be seen very easily from the Serb trenches above the city. The Serbs would wait for an old person to be visible, and then shoot them in the leg. When young people went to help them, the helpers would be killed. There was also a graveyard near to the Olympic Ice Stadium in which Torvill and Dean had won their gold medal in 1984 (*see* Plate 6.17). Many people were still being killed and burials were common (Plate 6.18). The Serbs then decided to kill people attending a funeral, and subsequently burials were restricted to a wooded area within the city. It was a very nasty war. The stadium was the base of the UN troops, and from here we would borrow the SAS armoured Land Rover when it was needed.

There were two social occasions never to be forgotten. Bosnia had an excellent reputation for classical music and even in the middle of the war classical concerts were still happening. They were different in two ways. The tickets were small – 5 × 8cm in size – as paper was extremely valuable, and the orchestra was made up of ladies and old men. All the young men were in the army. Despite the noise from occasional shelling, it was quite marvellous. As there was no street lighting it was possible to walk around relatively safely on moonless nights and on our last night Zjelka and her colleagues invited us all to her house, situated on a hill overlooking the city, for a farewell drink. And then to our great embarrassment, but heartfelt thanks, she produced a superb meal. There was hardly any food in the city, and how she managed it we never did discover. I was able to repay a very small part of her generosity when she visited us in England some ten years after the war finished.

And so after two weeks, one quiet and one very busy, we returned to the airfield. There I met and talked to a Danish colonel, who was returning home. He had tried to intervene with his command to stop the Srebrenica massacre but this was against the rules of engagement and as a result he had been sent home. Understandably he was a very bitter and disillusioned man. These were the same rules that allowed the Serbs to steal all our medical equipment, whilst the Italian soldiers looked on and could do nothing. At least the rules were changed soon afterwards.

And then we embarked in the flights home, firstly in the RAF Hercules and then via Rome with no problems. A few days off to recover physically and mentally would have been ideal, but we were all back at work the next day. My sincere thanks to the team. They performed brilliantly and we finished up as closer friends and colleagues. I know that some took a while to return to normality, and some are still conscious of the stress that the visit caused them. But I had become addicted to working in war zones, and when I was offered the opportunity of returning in October of the same year, the only problem was organising the time off from my NHS hospital. By moving my holidays around with the help of my colleagues, I did clear two weeks and three weekends. Looking back, I do not think that I saw much of my family that year.

For this second trip the list of people who would be most useful had changed as UK-Med had received our feedback and that from other visiting teams. The nursing there was excellent, and the only problems had arisen because of the lack of equipment. The general anaesthesia was also excellent, and our anaesthetists could help with the lack of brachial block anaesthetics. There was an MSF physiotherapist remaining on a longer-term basis. It was therefore agreed that one plastic surgeon, one anaesthetist and two ophthalmic surgeons would make up the team, and they would be accompanied by the same BBC TV team as on the first trip.

In mid-October we repeated the journey, again using Maybe Airlines. Back in June the RAF had got into trouble with the Foreign Office for putting their unofficial stamp in our passports, and so of course they repeated the offence in October. Well done the RAF! There is no stamp in my passports of which I am more proud.

The state of Sarajevo and its buildings had worsened and it was again a depressing place to be (*see* Plate 6.19). We were met by Dr John Navein, who although a qualified military GP (to the SAS) had taken on the post of logistician, and we settled into the same house that I had stayed in previously. And then on the next day we went to the University Hospital, where the welcome was utterly different from my previous visit. I suggested to Dr Hujic that I should do a clinic to select some patients. He smiled and we went onto the ward. Knowing that I was coming back, he had already selected the patients and the ward was full. The only change was that a somewhat elderly Bosniak plastic surgeon had managed to transfer from Banja Luka in the north, presumably through the tunnel, as Sarajevo was still surrounded by the Serbs.

With the help of the new anaesthetist, I started operating on the patient in one corner of the ward, and as the days progressed worked my way around the others. There were two of my old patients who had come for further work, including a young boy with very severe injuries to both arms and his body. He became the star of the TV programmes that followed. The only difference was that this time there were some burned patients, including a very badly burned child who unfortunately died. Burns had become more common as somehow gas was now available for cooking, but not officially for heating. The problem was that it had no smell, and lighting a cigarette with escaped gas in the room caused several explosions. I remember one day we were operating and there was a large explosion outside. The previous days after our arrival had been very much quieter than it had been in June, and the anaesthetist had not had the same experience as the rest of us. He disappeared rapidly into a corner. The local surgeons asked him if he was OK, and when he said that he was uninjured, their response was, 'What are you doing down there then?'

The social life included meals and excellent wine paid for by the British Ambassador in a local hotel, and visits to the flat of Mr and Mrs Kurtagic. Nadja, whom I had met on my June visit, was again our contact at the Ministry of Health. We also had walks around the city at night with the local anaesthetists and an excellent evening in our house, when John Navein invited some of his old SAS colleagues for a drink or two – or perhaps a few more!

I did have one severe sadness. During my June visit I had met a young dentist who had been shot through one hand some months previously. This had been patched up at the time, but her career as a dentist was finished without a major reconstruction. She needed two artificial joints to give her two worst affected fingers the possibility of working. These joints were not available at the time, but when I knew that I would be returning, I brought with me the necessary silicone joints, which had been very kindly donated by Smith & Nephew Ltd. I asked her anaesthetic friends to organise for me to see her and arrange the operation. They said that she had become severely depressed and was refusing any help. What a tragedy, and no doubt one of many during the long war, but it still upsets me.

We were extremely lucky with the weather on this visit. October can be the start of very cold winters in Bosnia, but we left before the temperatures dropped. In the previous winters people would spend long hours in bed or burn wooden furniture to keep warm, and after four years of war there was not much furniture left in most houses. Eventually the war finished in December 1995 with the signing of the Paris Agreement.

I was delighted to be invited by UK-Med to return to Bosnia in September 1996 with my wife Vivian. UK-Med had been funded by the governments of Britain and the United States and I can only think it must have had some money left over. The plan was to have a memorial dinner in the city hall for the volunteers and for the local medical staff. It was a marvellous occasion, and there were speeches both by the Bosnians and by us, expressing our thanks for the welcome that we had received, which included one by me. We were each then presented with a large bronze medal, and mine still adorns my wall. I thought it was a long way to go for the award only. Vivian had to return home to work, but I had managed to arrange two more weeks of leave from the NHS, and with local agreement and my thanks to my colleages at home, I stayed on to operate.

Plastic Surgery in Wars, Disasters and Civilian Life

The pattern of surgery had changed. The city was no longer surrounded and the local population was returning to the fields to farm. A mine-clearance programme had started but there were still mines in abundance, causing what was for me a different form of injury from anything that I had previously treated. Using basic principles, I rapidly learned to help people by producing good stumps so that artificial legs could be fitted. During the war a workshop had been set up to make artificial legs from spare parts obtained from the local rubbish dump. They were very effective but not very cosmetic.

There was one very interesting patient whom I have already mentioned in Chapter 5. It would have been possible to produce a stump, but because of the amount of tissue that had been blown off, this would have needed the limb to be shortened above the knee, causing a considerable extra loss of function. Using the microsurgical skills that I had learned in Australia, it was possible to move part of the patient's skin and tissues from his back and thus to keep his functional knee. An ex-military trainee of mine was in charge of the UN hospital outside Sarajevo, and he persuaded his commanding officer that his help was necessary as my assistant. This worked, and so did the microvascular flap. This was a very early, if not the first, example of the military and civilians working together in a war zone, and I am delighted to say it has now become normal practice.

We stayed with the Kurtagics on this visit, and met again many colleagues with whom I had worked during the war. We could also walk around both in the city and on the local hills. We went up to the Serb trenches above the Holiday Inn (*see* Plate 6.20), and I picked up some bullet cases. I have them still, and they do bring back memories.

What is the future for Bosnia? The situation there had been less than ideal for centuries and although it was improving, matters were made far worse by the war. There had been intermarriages between Serbs and Bosnians, which nearly all broke down, and Zjelka, one of my anaesthetic friends in Sarajevo, supported Bosnia, but her sister supported Serbia and had moved away. There are no clear origins for the war. Certainly there had been religious, political and economic differences held under control by President Tito for many years. The best summary that I have read is the book by Noel Malcolm, *Bosnia – A Short History*.

The present situation remains far from ideal. Politically there is a mix of Muslim Bosniaks and Orthodox Serbs. The latter are in a minority and are less than happy. The Serbs proclaimed their area as the independent country Srpska, which comprised about 30 per cent of the country by population. Srpska is not recognised by any country in the world except Serbia, which signed a Special Ties Agreement in 2006. Religion is also split with 50 per cent of the population Muslim, 30 per cent Orthodox Christians and 15 per cent, mostly of Croatian origin, Roman Catholic. Several of the past leaders have been indicted at the War Crimes Tribunal in The Hague and are now either dead or in prison.

After those depressing paragraphs I was delighted to revisit the country in October 2001 as a visiting professor at the First Bosnian Plastic Surgery Conference. This time I somehow kept out of the operating theatres. Vivian and I again stayed with the Kurtagics and discovered more of their history. The husband, Effe (Ephraim), had been the major foreign correspondent for Yugonews, and had met an incredible array of people including Stalin and most of the Russian heads of state since. They had owned a large house in Belgrade, which was confiscated when Bosnia broke away. They still had a country house in Mali Ston in Croatia, which they had managed to keep, and we have also stayed there with them and their daughter Sanja.

Some rebuilding had started in Sarajevo, of which the graveyard was an example (*see* Plate 6.21).

Azerbaijan, 1988–1994

It is ironic that as I am writing this (in 2020) the Armenian Azerbaijani War is raging once more.

Nagorno-Karabakh is an area in the south-west of Azerbaijan. In the 1980s the majority of people living there were Armenians who voted for the area to become independent as the Republic of Artsakh, and part of Armenia. This move was rejected by Azerbaijan. A process of ethnic cleansing therefore started slowly in 1988, but increased in the early 1990s until a ceasefire was agreed in 1994. By that time 700,000 Azeris had been moved out of Nagorno-Karabakh into Azerbaijan and 230,000 Armenians had been moved out of Azerbaijan to Armenia. During the war the total reported deaths and injuries for the Azeris were 25,000 and 50,000 respectively, and for the Armenians 8,000 and 20,000.

The vast majority of the Azeris who had been displaced were living in three tented camps or in disused railway carriages in the south-west of the country. One of the problems was that these people were IDPs (Internally Displaced Persons) and therefore not refugees, which would have brought them under the umbrella of the United Nations. Another problem was that in 1994 Azerbaijan was a very poor country. It had oil (the earliest

Plastic Surgery in Wars, Disasters and Civilian Life

reports of oil gushing out of the rocks date to the third and fourth centuries AD), but no way of shipping it out to sell. The conditions in the camps were very poor (*see* Plate 6.22) and various countries offered help. The Norwegians, for instance, supported education, and the British medical care.

The Leonard Cheshire Department of Conflict Recovery at University College, London, under the leadership of Professor Colonel Jim Ryan, was organising the British response. In the camps there was one young English GP and some nurses giving day-to-day care. It had become apparent that specialist care was also needed, and particularly surgery. In the capital, Baku, there was a very large ex-Russian hospital. Because of the severe poverty of most of the population this hospital was almost empty. There were two general surgeons working there and Jim Ryan had funded the treatment of some patients from the camps. As it became clearer that specialist surgery was required, plastic and orthopaedic surgeons from the United Kingdom were funded to travel out, visit the encampments to select patients, and then to operate in the hospital. Living in a camp of that size is dangerous, especially for young children. The family parties were large and the poor cooking and heating facilities were causing numerous accidents including burns.

My first two-week visit was in 1998. The rather ancient plane with no entertainment of any kind arrived to the minute at Baku airport, where I was met by our interpreter Homa and taken to the hotel. The next morning we drove on an interesting, mainly dirt, road through land that was mostly flat and with lakes often on both sides for nearly 200 miles to the largest IDP camp very close to the Iranian border. We were met by the British GP stationed there and did an out-patient clinic of patients he thought might be appropriate. Most of them were children with old injuries, and certainly several would benefit from surgery, particularly for relieving scar contractures. How the transfers or organisation happened I do not know, but the next morning in Baku my patients had been admitted and were ready for surgery. The two local general surgeons were both delightful and competent, and operated with me for the rest of the time. Competent was not, however, a word that could be used of the anaesthetist, and at one point I had to take over the anaesthetic to keep a young child alive. My African experience was very useful. With some touring around the beautiful old city in the evenings, and the company of the two surgeons who took me to various places, we passed a very useful and pleasant two weeks. I am definitely not a foodie but the final farewell meal of barbecued sturgeon lives on in my memory.

After discussion with Jim Ryan, it was agreed that I would return for a further two weeks the following year, and could also invite an anaesthatist to come as well. Needless to say my first choice was my old colleague Richard Bunsell, and being Richard, he immediately said yes. Jim also thought that he would come himself to see what was happening and to make plans for the future. From a surgical point of view, the weeks were very similar, but this time it was an enormous relief to be able to trust the anaesthetist. The social life also improved, and I remember particularly a visit to a meeting where there was local singing and dancing, which the two local surgeons joined in. On my third visit in 2000 I was accompanied by Vivian, who very much enjoyed the old town. Sadly, soon afterwards, support from the Leonard Cheshire Foundation ended. I did not return to the country until 2019, when Vivian and I joined a Wild Frontiers tour of the three countries. We started in Azerbaijan, and it was a country that neither of us recognised except by its portrayal in the Bond film 'The World is not Enough'. It now has oil flowing out through a new pipeline and is a relatively rich country with some magnificent new buildings, better shops and, according to our guide, improvements for all the population. We then went on to Georgia and then to Armenia. There, there was no mention of the Azerbaijan war, only of the Turkish genocide. Recalling conditions in the camps, I felt uncomfortable when we were in Armenia. Given the enormous differences in race, religion and language, unfortunately I have serious doubts of any long-lasting peace in the area.

Kosovo
Between 1998 and 1999 there was fighting between the Serbs and the Kosovans. The problems had been almost identical to the situation in Nagorno-Karabakh. Kosovo had been part of Yugoslavia, and on the break-up of that country became part of Serbia. The Serbs were particularly attached to the area as there was evidence that their religion had started there, and certainly there were several ancient monasteries and nunneries in the countryside. The major problem was that the land was ocupied by a people whose origin, language and religion were Albanian, and they were in a large majority. They also claimed that they had been persecuted, and this I was to discover was accurate.

After the Plastic Surgery Conference in Sarajevo in 2001, we had planned to visit Tom and Fi Morrison in Pristina, the capital of Kosovo.

The Morrisons were long-standing friends of ours from Buckinghamshire. Tom is an internationally recognised agricultural economist, and he had taken a posting from the World Bank to live in Kosovo with his wife for a year to ensure the appropriate use of the donations that had been given to the country, and to develop agricultural policies. By chance, at the conference in Sarajevo I had met Violeta and Sender Zatriqi, who were Kosovan surgeons, and they had asked me to visit them and their hospital in Pristina. Vivian and I took a bus for the 160-mile journey from Sarajevo through Montenegro, just bypassing Albania, to Pristina, an interesting journey in itself. We were met by Tom and Fi and stayed with them for a week. During the week we met Violeta and Sender and various colleagues on several occasions, and visited the hospital. We discovered that when the Serbs moved out, they had completely stripped the hospital of all its equipment. For several years previously it had also been the case that a doctor of Albanian background could not work in a hospital or a clinic, and that Albanian surgeons, as their only way of working, had been operating in their own garages, facing possible persecution at any time.

When we visited, some basic equipment had been donated internationally and the doctors, although wishing for further training, had started working again. Because of the lack of facilities during the conflict, only very poor emergency surgery had been available, and there were therefore many patients needing secondary work. Two Swedish surgeons had offered their help and for some years made various short visits to perform surgery.

The Morrisons very kindly lent us their car and Vivian and I did some touring through the stunningly attractive countryside and the second city, Prizren. With the Morrisons we also visited a monastery and a nunnery, which were well guarded by UN soldiers, and both of which were stunning. We were strongly welcomed and given marvellous tours. We were talking to the Prior in the garden of one of them when there was a very loud explosion outside the wall. The Prior and I, both used to such bangs, carried on our conversation without a break. Vivian and the Morrisons all jumpoed and looked somewhat worried. I explained the Sarajevo philosophy that if you hear a large bang and are not injured – why worry!

What astonished both Vivian and I was that no other friends, nor even their own children, had taken the opportunity of their generosity to visit the Morrisons during their year in the country. After this visit I arranged

Medical Care in Disasters and Wars

for Violeta, the plastic surgeon, to have a educational short visit to England.

In 2007, much to my surprise, I had an invitation from Violeta to be the keynote speaker at an international conference on plastic surgery and burns that she had organised. Truly she was a lady of spirit. Vivian and I very happily returned and stayed with a neighbour of the Zatriqis. The conference at which I was speaking changed somewhat unexpectedly in that I was also demonstrating surgery by closed link television from the hospital. The University kindly gave me the title of Professor of Surgery for my minor efforts.

My last war was a much more minor effort on my part, but it is always encouraging to see a country pulling itself up again after a disaster or war, and this was happening in Pristina when we revisited in 2007, though not, I understand, in some enclaves of the country where the Serbs were still living in an unhappy state and seeking independence.

During the Kosovan hostilities 8,600 Albanian Kosovans, 1,800 Serbs, 460 other races including Roma and Bosniaks, and two US peacekeeping soldiers were killed. And in 2020 some of the Kosovan leaders from the war period were in The Hague to face a war crimes court.

Postscript

The most important change that I have seen, and perhaps been a little responsible for, over the twenty years covered by these four wars is that military and civilian teams started working together. This is of enormous benefit to both. The military have medical personnel and unusual skills such as air transport for both patients and staff. They also have tented hospitals packed and ready to go. The civilian organisations can send larger numbers of senior consultants and nurses, adding to the general military capabilities.

In summary, I think that any experience is useful as it is really difficult to train for the one unique situation that might occur out of the thousand possibilities. My previous work in developing countries I found extremely valuable.

The Roman poet Ovid had the most valid thoughts on disasters and wars 2000 years ago:

Semper faecubus summus – Sole profundo variat.
(We are always in the shit – Only the depth varies.)

To add to the confusion I can add: 'And the Press are always with us.'

Chapter 7

Motor Racing Track Doctor

During the summer of 1975 when I was working at Cheltenham General Hospital, I was doing a routine general surgical out-patient clinic. As I finished each patient, I would go to the door to show them out and call for the next patient on the list. I noticed a man who had not moved, and at the end of the clinic when I had seen everybody on my list, he was still there. He came over and asked if he could have a word. 'Are you doing anything this weekend?' Slightly suspicious I asked, 'Why?'

He told me he was an organiser of the Prescott Hill Climb, and they were desperate for a doctor or the meeting that weekend of the Bugatti Owners' Club would have to be cancelled. He then told me what was needed, and that I would be provided with lunch and a bottle of champagne. The latter made the decision easier! I signed up and on the Saturday arrived at the famous hill climb site to find a couple of first aiders and an ancient ambulance in attendance. A hill climb consists of a timed ascent of each car in order up a steep and twisting track. It was really an event left over from the 1920s when cars had far less power than today's average mini. I admired the old cars and then parked half-way up the track. The good news was that there were no crashes, and I had nothing to do to earn my lunch and champagne.

I subsequently did two further meetings there, and on one was accompanied by Vivian. On that occasion I took my very rare Aston Martin, which attracted almost as much attention as the beautiful Bugattis and Ferraris that were competing.

That was the start of my career as a track doctor, though I did no more until I was appointed to Stoke Mandeville Hospital, which is 20 miles south of the renowned Silverstone race track. I remember becoming involved again through the Aston Martin Owners' Club (AMOC). Many of the small clubs were often short of medical officers and I covered several weekend events for various clubs including AMOC, the Vintage Sports Car Club and the 750 Club. It was rare not to have to do some work, but luckily, whether I was on my own or had paramedics and first aiders in support, nothing too serious happened at any of the events. These small events had one major advantage in that there were rarely any spectators who could be injured. I do, however, remember one AMOC meeting where a car lost a wheel, which went bouncing down the track, and then off the track aiming directly at one spectator. For some unexplained reason he just stood there until it hit him in the chest and flattened him – luckily, leaving him with no more than some sore ribs, and no doubt later a bruise.

I slowly worked my way up through the ranks and the first major meetings that I covered included six years at the Coy's Historic Festival. This was the primary event in the UK for old cars and had a large number of cars and also spectators. I found out about the medical back-up required for such events. There was (and is) a superb medical centre at Silverstone, with two intensive care admission bays, two operating theatres and even a small emergency burn unit as well as a radiography department. There were five or six doctors and a good support staff on site. For one of the Coy's Festivals we were short of an orthopaedic surgeon, and I recruited one of my fellow consultants from Stoke Mandeville, Bernard McElroy. I was showing him around, and in the paddock waiting to go onto the track for the first race were some twenty old and beautiful Ferraris, worth about £1 million each. 'They are surely not going to race these, are they?' said Bernie. My reply was, 'You wait and see.' They do, of course, race these magnificent cars, but they also try very hard to avoid damage to their own car or any other car.

A few years later I was asked to join the medical team for the Formula 1 weekend at Silverstone. This team consisted of forty-three surgeons, anaesthetists, accident doctors, a radiologist and two other long-term volunteers. One of these was an obstetrician and the other a VD doctor, and there was the suspicion that the latter might be of more use to the drivers than the rest of us! There were also eight paramedics, four theatre sisters, a fast medical response car, four ambulances and a helicopter. On race days the medical centre was fully staffed, the senior doctor and a paramedic were in the fast response car, there were two doctors on the pit wall (myself as the burn expert and one other), and a doctor with a rescue crew positioned every quarter of a mile around the track. Clearly the drivers deserve the best possible care, but the real worry are the spectators, who at Silverstone can number over 140,000 on race days. During the Le Mans 24-hour race in 1955 a car flew off the track and into the spectators, killing eighty-four and injuring more than a hundred. This was the background to the safety precautions at the track and the medical facilities on site.

Formula 1 had long had a poor reputation for safety. I remember John Surtees telling me that 50 per cent of the drivers he had raced against had been killed. On discussing this with Jackie Stewart, he said that a few years later, when he was racing, the figure had improved to 33 per cent. Jackie, with the senior medical officer at the time, Professor Sid Watkins, had made real and successful efforts to improve safety over several years, and these efforts have been recorded in Sid's books *Life at the Limit* and *Beyond the Limit*. When I was involved, the local hospital facilities were at Northampton General Hospital for most accidents, Stoke Mandeville for burns and spinal injuries, and the John Radcliffe at Oxford for neurosurgery, and all were inspected prior to each meeting.

At the Grand Prix of 1999 Michael Schumacher had a serious crash at Stowe corner and broke his right leg. He was looked after by Bernie McElroy, the orthopaedic consultant from Stoke Mandeville, who had by this time become a regular member of the team. Bernie sent him to a colleague at Northampton, who operated and plated his leg. Afterwards Ferrari gave the Northampton consultant a car, and needless to say Bernie was considerably upset!

I had various especially interesting experiences over the years. On one practice day the Duke of Kent, who was patron of the British Racing Drivers' Club (BRDC), and himself a keen motorist, was walking down the pit lane towards me. I stepped out in front of him, but with my hat and earphones he clearly did not recognise me instantly. A few steps further and recognition came to him. 'Hello Anthony – good to see you.' He then introduced me to Max Mosley from the BRDC, his daughter Lady Helen Taylor and her husband Timothy. He asked me if I was busy, to which the answer was no. 'Then come along with us.' And with them I went into all the pits and talked to several drivers, including Michael Schumacher, with whom I had several interesting minutes of conversation.

The second memorable occasion was in the year 2000, when the usual June date of the British Grand Prix had been rearranged to April, for unknown reasons. That week it had poured with rain and in the spectator car park on qualifying day there was chaos, with many cars stuck in the mud. Cars were therefore banned for race day. I was walking around in the starting grid area and came across Bernie Ecclestone, the guru of Formula 1 at the time, and we struck up a conversation. The chaos caused by the rain came up and I asked him if we were going to hold the race at

Christmas the following year. I do not think that he was amused, and several colleagues told me there would be no job for me the following year! But as Bernie used my joke later in a television interview, I thought that my job should be safe.

Another story about Bernie was that he always arrived by helicopter. One year the cloud base was so low that the helicopter could not fly, and he arrived at the main gate by car, but without a ticket. The man at the gate, even after he was told whom he was talking to, still would not let him in until his supervisor appeared. Very interestingly, Bernie congratulated the gateman for sticking to the rules and we were all impressed.

Another interesting encounter was with Frankie Dettori and Arnold Schwarzenegger. They had been taken around the starting grid and I was asked to look after them on the pit wall for the race. Frankie was bouncing up and down with excitement though Arnie looked extremely bored.

In return for our services, we were offered accommodation or travel expenses and a guest ticket. One year we were told that the guest ticket was not on offer, but were smartly told that in that case, we would have to charge the full commercial rate of £2,000 each. The tickets arrived in the next post! We were also provided with a set of flameproof racing overalls every three or four years. I had the idea of collecting the signatures of the drivers on mine. The first set I kept for F1 World champions – of which I have sixteen, going back to the late Phil Hill, the champion in 1978. I am only missing four recent champions and one older champion, Kimi Raikonen. The second set has the signature of British Formula 1 drivers.

During my time with Formula 1, the requirement for the Advanced Trauma Life Support (ATLS) qualification was introduced. Courses were organised yearly at Silverstone, directed by an ex-trainee of mine, Nick James. We were offered very preferential rates. I am pleased to say that I passed, but unfortunately two of my senior consultant colleagues who had been regular track doctors failed and that was the end of F1 for them. The exam had to be repeated every four years, and on my third attempt they were obviously fed up with me, and through the good offices of Dr Ian Roberts, who later became the senior F1 doctor, they made me an instructor candidate. I followed this up, was approved and have now instructed on more than a hundred courses throughout the country. The course at Silverstone included an evening session of indoor karting. With sixteen track doctors and paramedics, it was not surprisingly very competitive. All went well until one year Dr David Cranston, the senior Silverstone doctor, crashed and broke three ribs. We were also given the option

Motor Racing Track Doctor

of another different session and I did the four-wheel off-road course and drove a Formula Junior single-seater around a shortened course for an afternoon.

During my ten years in Formula 1 I did not have to look after any drivers, but tended to several of the pit crews with minor injuries.

When we moved to the Isle of Wight in 2001, I continued with Formula 1 for some years and also covered meetings at Thruxton and Brands Hatch. I also contacted the Goodwood Motor Racing circuit. There is an interesting history to Goodwood. It lies within the estate of the 11th Duke of Richmond (who is also confusingly known as the Earl of March) and is based around Goodwood House. The motor racing is in two parts, a race circuit and a hill climb. The hill climb was first run in 1936 for the Lancia Car Club and at some time afterwards fell into disuse. In 1993 it was revived as the 'Festival of Speed', which was a seriously competitive event. In 2000 there was a fatal accident when a driver and a marshal were killed, and a second marshal lost both legs. This was thought to have been caused by the driver having a heart attack. Over time, and with the introduction of Formula 1 cars to the event, it has become much less competitive, and is more of a demonstration of cars and drivers, although timing does still occur for the few who wish to race.

The hill climb track starts on the flat past the house with a long right-hand bend, and this is where most of the spectators are situated in stands or wherever they can find a vantage point. There is then Molecomb, a vicious left-hand bend with an adverse camber which catches out many drivers who finish up in the straw bales. The hill starts just beyond that corner and close to a flint wall. The stretch to the finish is relatively straight. The cars are sent up in batches and after finishing they park up until the batch is complete, after which they all return down the hill to the paddocks, in theory slowly.

The motor racing circuit was opened in 1948 and used until 1966, when it was closed. In a Formula 1 race (not part of the championship) Stirling Moss crashed his Lotus car here and was in a coma for a month in the Atkinson Morley Neurology Hospital. In 1998 the track was reopened with a Revival Meeting. This has been held every year since and is restricted to cars built before 1966. As well as old cars, the dress code for the spectators and the marshals is ideally also vintage, and the only people in modern flame-resistant clothes are the drivers and the medical and ambulance teams.

Following my application, Jay Simson, who was a general surgeon at Chichester Hospital and also the senior medical officer at Goodwood, invited me along to my first meeting in 2001. It was a very different set-up from Silverstone. There was a first aid room and an ambulance, which was shared between the drivers and the spectators. There were six or eight doctors, many of whom had done motor race doctoring for some years. Four or five were surgeons, one or two anaesthetists and the remainder GPs. There were no formal checks on qualifications, and I never heard ATLS mentioned. In 2001 there were far fewer spectators than at Silverstone, but the numbers quite rapidly increased over the years and had reached up to 70,000 a day by 2012. In the beginning first aid for the spectators was provided by St John Ambulance volunteers, with the track doctors helping when required. As the numbers increased, spectator care became more professional. The track doctors were unpaid, but through the generosity of Jay and Annie Simson we were accommodated in their house, where there was a party to remember on the Saturday night. As the years progressed, Jay gave up the organisation and it became professional. The track doctors began to have problems with their insurance cover for medical work, and we were then paid. I carried on until 2012, by which time I was the only one of the old crew still volunteering (or by then getting paid). The pleasure was being slowly removed, and I had had enough. The increasing lack of experience in the team also began to worry me, as the accident rate with old drivers in old cars on the very fast but less well designed course was far higher than at Silverstone.

I much preferred the Festival of Speed, where I was normally situated at the busiest corner at Molecomb. When off duty, we were not allowed to ride up in a competitor's car, but we could have a ride up in the course car which followed up the last of each batch. We could then persuade one of the drivers to give us a lift down the hill and back to the paddocks. The theory was that they drove slowly back down the hill, but with a doctor in the car that did not seem to happen! Over the years I cadged lifts from several drivers, who included two British Le Mans winners, Derek Bell and Andy Wallace. Once I came down in a 100-year-old Mercedes with wooden wheels at 60mph, and another time in a Lola Chevrolet T163 with the American driver John Bell. The engine on this car produced 950bhp and the car accelerated from 0–60mph in 2 seconds. After that I had a stiff neck for a week! At the top of the hill I had the opportunity of getting the signatures of more F1 winning drivers on my racing overalls, as well as talking with Lord March, Jacques Villeneuve, Stirling Moss and John Surtees, Murray Walker and Steve Rider, the TV commentator.

I also talked to Lewis Hamilton, Jensen Button, Alan Jones, John Surtees and several other drivers as they gave me their autographs. I remember discussing his motor-cycle with somebody I did not recognise at all and noticed several people lined up with autograph books waiting for us to finish. He clearly saw that I had not a clue who he was, and was only interested in his bike, and he became much more relaxed. I was told afterwards that he was Ewan McGregor, the actor.

There were some serious accidents. The worst whilst I was there was at Molecomb corner. A German former motor-cycle and sidecar world champion was doing a demonstration run up the hill. He was about 80 years old and we learned later that his son had tried to persuade him not to do it. Very tragically in the crash he fractured his spine, and his sidecar passenger, also elderly, had serious injuries to his chest, with multiple fractured ribs and pneumothoraces on both sides.

Another motor-cyclist also crashed at Molecomb just in front of me, and was unconscious and not breathing. The problem with motor-cyclists is removing the crash helmet, or at least the visor, so that oxygen can be given with a mask and bag. This we did and he rapidly returned to his normal state of mind and body. The following year he found me, and gave me a £10 note to buy a drink for myself and the colleague who had been with me!

In another year a well known Formula 1 world champion came off on the same corner. He was not obviously injured and wanted the marshals to push his car clear so that he could continue. The rule was, and is, that any driver involved in a crash must be checked by a doctor. We had a gentle discussion, with me eventually laying down the law. I found nothing wrong with him, and he continued up the hill. He knew that the rule is that a doctor has the right to instantly suspend a racing licence at any time.

On the race track for the Revival Meeting there were four accidents that I remember vividly. Two of these occurred at Madgwick corner, which was where Stirling Moss had had his disastrous accident. The old cars were not fitted with seat belts, and an elderly driver had been thrown out of his car and was clearly unconscious. He was bleeding profusely in his mouth which made it impossible to use the bag and mask to give him oxygen. At this point the medical car with an anaesthetist arrived. Two of us used mobile suckers to try to remove the blood without success, and Dr Gary Smith, an intensive care anaesthetist from Portsmouth, managed to do a blind intubation to put a tube into his trachea. Without a doubt his brilliance saved the driver's life. We discovered later that the driver had also fractured the base of his skull, and had several other injuries. He was in hospital for three months and lost one eye. The next year he came back to thank all those who had worked on him.

At the same corner a driver hit the bank, severely damaging both his car and himself. He was trapped in the car. The marshals were quickly there with fire extinguishers, which enabled the specialist marshals to begin to cut him out. As with all car owners, the driver was much more upset that his car was being torn apart than about his injuries. However, when he was extracted, it was obvious to him that both his legs were at right angles to where they should have been. When the driver saw his legs, he commented that his wife had been trying to persuade him to give up racing for some time, and he could now see why. He also had a severe dislocation of one ankle, which was reduced, and his legs straightened, before being put in the ambulance.

The next two accidents were not serious, but involved the same driver in the same car at the same place – Lavant Corner – in succeeding years. This corner is the steepest on the track, with a good gravel run-off area, and although accidents there are common they are normally minor. The driver on both occasions was a friend of mine, Anthony Goddard from the Isle of Wight. As he stepped out of his Formula Junior car, which was stuck in the gravel, he took one look at me and asked, 'What the hell are you doing here?' The next year his comment in the identical situation was, 'Not you again – I don't believe it!' And, I will admit, neither did I.

Goodwood was overall a marvellous experience. Old cars were and are a passion of mine, and although it is interesting to talk to Formula 1 and Le Mans drivers, the modern cars are far less appealing. Jay and Annie Simson and the team of doctors who included Jonathan Botting and Kate Gill were great fun and it was excellent to work with them. At the Revival Meeting there was a special car park for anyone who came with a pre-1966 car. I took my 1960 Daimler V8 SP250 sports car almost every year. One year somebody whom I had never met was inspecting my car when he noticed that I had a wheel trim missing. He had previously owned the same model so he took my address and sent me the wheel trim that he had left in his garage as a gift! There is an amazing camaraderie amongst old car owners.

During my twelve years as a track doctor at Goodwood, and through connections that I made, I was asked to attend various meetings at

Thruxton, which was the other track relatively near to the Isle of Wight, a Touring Car championship weekend at Brands Hatch, and one further meeting at the Prescott Hill Climb.

Cars and not motorbikes were my interest, but through the kindness of Peter Chapman, an old patient of mine who had become a trustee of my medical research charity, I was invited for several years to watch the British Motor-Cycle Grand Prix at Donington. Peter was a friend and old racing colleague of Tom Wheatcroft, who owned Donington, and who had a marvellous Formula 1 car museum there. Tom gave us a personal guided tour, and at the same time told us the background to his life, which was fascinating. There was no family money and when he was leaving school his father asked him whether he wanted to work on a farm or on building sites. Tom asked which job would pay better and was told that construction offered a few shillings a week more. That had obviously made the decision easier, and Tom went on to become an extremely wealthy man within the building industry.

From somewhere also came an invitation to be a track doctor at the Isle of Man TT races. This was not my interest, and the prospect of having to deal psychologically with an average of two deaths a year would not have been easy, and so I refused the offer. They must have been short as the offer was repeated yearly for ten years – as was my refusal.

In summary, being a track doctor over a span of nearly forty years was an interesting addition to my medical work, and I made some good friends. I was never involved in a track fatality, for which I am thankful. They will remain nameless, but I did look after several well-known drivers either before or after their Formula 1 or Indycar careers, but thankfully their accidents and immediate care were not shown on television.

Chapter 8

St John Ambulance

The black and white uniforms of St John Ambulance had often been in the background at different times of my career. I knew that they were voluntary first aid workers but little else about the organisation. My first aid I had learned in the Scouts. When I was a registrar in Birmingham, I had been asked to examine St John people for their qualifying examination. Not knowing what they were expected to know, and not being given any instructions, made this a difficult job. It was all right for the first two or three, but after twenty in an afternoon it became a little boring asking the same questions. But it was then a paid job!

Thirty years later, just before leaving Stoke Mandeville, I was asked to be the examiner at the Buckinghamshire County St John cadet competition. For an unknown reason I accepted. This time what was required was more clearly stated, and I enjoyed the evening. The St John County Medical Officer asked me if I would be interested in joining him and helping. I explained that I was in my last few months in Buckinghamshire and would then be moving to the Isle of Wight. He said he was sure that I would be very welcome to help there. I cannot now remember why, but when I arrived on the Isle of Wight I did contact St John, and was immediately put on the County St John council.

An introduction to the very complicated organisation would be sensible at this stage. And I am still learning about the organisation more than twenty years later. Its origin dates back before 1080, at which time a hospital had been established in Jerusalem to care for sick pilgrims. The religious order that ran it had by 1113 become known as the Hospitallers. After the Crusades, the Hospitallers took on a military role and became the Knights of the Order of St John of Jerusalem. When Palestine was captured by the Muslims in 1291, the order moved to Cyprus, and then in 1309 went to Rhodes, where it remained until 1522, when again, following capture of the island by the Muslims, the order moved to Malta. The original headquarters are still in Valetta, virtually unchanged. The order still has headquarters in Rome and is called the Sovereign Military

Hospitaller Order of St John of Jerusalem, of Rhodes and of Malta. In the 1140s the English headquarters were established in the Priory in Clerkenwell, and this remained until Henry VIII dissolved all Roman Catholic churches, and Queen Elizabeth I permanently dissolved the Order.

As a replacement, the Most Venerable Order of the Hospital of St John of Jerusalem, as it was properly called, was established in England and granted a royal charter by Queen Victoria in 1888. It established the St John Eye Hospital in Jerusalem and the St John Ambulance Brigade. It is now known as the Order of St John and is a Christian order, although since 1999 it has been open to persons of any faith or no faith.

The Brigade, which later became St John Ambulance, provided volunteers for the South African War and both world wars, where they acted as stretcher-bearers in the front line and had hospitals close to the fronts (*see* Plate 8.1). In 1908 it provided first aid for the Olympics in London, and its role has since continued for sporting and general events. In 1922 it set up cadet units for training young people between the ages of 11 and 18, and in 1987 the Badgers were established for children between 5 and 11.

The Priory since its establishment has been the basis of the charity and includes all of England and Wales and the Islands. Scotland broke away in 1908 and the equivalent organisation there is St Andrew's Ambulance. Still under the trusteeship of the Priory, St John Ambulance is administratively separate but closely linked, and its headquarters are next to the Priory building in London. It was originally organised on a county basis until 2015, when it became national.

The Order recommends to the Crown people for awards. These are at five levels. Level 1 was previously known as Serving Brother or Serving Sister until 2014, when it became Member; Level 2 is Officer; Level 3 is Commander; Level 4 is Knight or Dame; and Level 5 is Bailiff or Dame Grand Cross. Although it is a national award, the post-nominal letters are only used within the organisation and on gravestones, etc., and the titles of Knight and Dame are used in the same way. It is confusing, and even more so as the medals are worn on any uniform or formal dress when royalty or the equivalent are present.

The Ambulance has a separate system and gives awards, medals and bars for length of active service. This starts at twelve years for the medal, and bars for every five years of further active service. Sew-on badges are now also awarded for three, six and nine years of service prior to the first medal. There are ranks within the Ambulance for different levels of management, and also titles and different colour epaulettes for levels of training. These latter levels are Doctor (Red), Nurse (Grey) and Paramedic (Green). These three levels are called Health Care Professionals (HCP). Black epaulettes differentiate the other three levels, which are Ambulance Crew, Advanced First Aider and First Aider.

There also exists St John International, which oversees equivalent organisations in forty-one countries that were formerly part of the British Empire, and also the United States. At higher levels there are connections with St Andrew's Ambulance and the Red Cross. They jointly publish a First Aid Guide, which is now in its eleventh edition, and also meet at committee level twice a year.

On a day to day basis there used to be considerable rivalry between the Red Cross and St John Ambulance, since both were trying to attract work, but this ceased in 2020 when the Red Cross stopped doing duties at events in the United Kingdom. And if you are not now as confused as I am about St John, I have obviously failed!

Some months after I joined the local St John Council, an advertisement came around about a national conference for health care professionals. I went and whilst at this conference I met the medical advisers of both St John and the Red Cross. Both were about to retire, and they each suggested that I should apply for their post. Knowing very little about the organisations, there appeared to be little difference between them. As the St John post was to be vacant four months earlier, I went for that one. The medical adviser was a paid role based at the headquarters in London for two days a week. The role was both to advise the senior management and to work under the Chief Medical Officer. This latter was a volunteer post and normally occupied by a retired senior military medical officer. When I applied, Lieutenant General Bob Menzies was in post. He had been the Surgeon General, the most senior medic of all three services. I was appointed and arranged to work my two days contiguously, staying the night in London either at the Royal College of Surgeons or at the Royal Air Force Club. I did start to look around for a flat closer to St John HQ, but never bought one. The first thing that had to be altered was my contract. This stated that I had to retire at 65, which I had already reached. This was no problem, as St John for a few years had allowed all staff and volunteers to continue until they were unfit to work. The work was very administrative and included sitting on various committees. One useful job that I did was to proof-read the new *First Aid Guide for Treating the Homeless* that St John was producing. One of our team was John Newman, who was developing and introducing the new role of First Aid

Responder around the country. This was for senior St John first aiders in more rural parts of England who could respond rapidly to 999 calls and arrive some vital minutes before an ambulance. This has since been shown to be very useful, and John was subsequently awarded an MBE for his work. He also asked me if I would become a volunteer. He organised a group of senior St John volunteers whose role was to work with the Royal Protection Group of the Metropolitan Police and the Household Cavalry, providing first aid to the royal family and senior government ministers on all state occasions. These included Trooping the Colour, the State Opening of Parliament, the Armistice Day parade, the Order of the Garter, Royal Ascot and any state visits. I became a volunteer and went on Operation Try-out with the police and the cavalry in Norfolk. It was very interesting learning how to deal with very large horses jumping around with explosions and gunfire all around. I also found out how incredibly difficult it was to extract an injured person from a state carriage! During the next months I attended meetings in London and Scotland, gave a lecture on burn management at the annual Health Care Professionals' conference and was a judge at the national cadet competition. After some months in London, I realised that a lot of my day-to-day work could be done from home on the telephone and I suggested that I should do this. This would save me wasted time sitting at a desk on occasions doing very little, and also save St John some money as I would only charge for my time worked. This was turned down, not by Bob Menzies but by the administration, and I never did discover why. I have learned over the years that managers hate change – unless it is their idea. I therefore retired from the job but continued as a very active volunteer.

Looking back I wonder if I would have been happier with the Red Cross and its international role, but this role had not been mentioned and I think was at a different level.

My work on the island St John Council continued, and a lot of the work then at county level involved raising money. The Isle of Wight is a strange place. It was, and is, the second poorest county in Britain, with both high unemployment and a larger percentage of elderly residents than any other county. It is markedly divided between the well-off and the poor, and it was a difficult place to raise the money needed to keep the St John work active. Anyone trying to raise money there very soon learns that it is virtually impossible unless one can say that the money will be used on the island. Vivian is the expert fundraiser in our household, and she helped to organise as her first effort an evening meal at Haseley Manor, where the speaker was George Band, one of the 1953 Everest team. Since then she has organised, with a little help from me and with meals prepared by members of the charities involved, five other such lunches or evenings which have raised money for St John and the island scouts. These talks have been by Professor Charles Higham, an old Cambridge friend of mine, on the Angkor community of south-east Asia, by HRH the Duke of Kent, by Lord Fowler, by Alan Titchmarsh and by Sir Ben Ainslie. All were excellent, fully attended and raised several thousand pounds each.

With my new volunteer hat on, I was made Deputy County Surgeon and given my black and white uniform. There are national guidelines for medical and first aid cover at sporting events which are in the Green Guide, and for non-sporting events which are in the Purple Guide. In the 2000s St John covered a large range of events on the island, of which the large ones requiring medical cover and not first aid only were the two pop music festivals, the Cowes fireworks, the Garlic Festival, Motor-Cross and the Proms in the Park at Osborne House. I covered the last three of these for several years, and managed to avoid the pop festivals, as my hearing was already beginning to fail and I would not have been able to talk to any patient with the noise level expected. Our Lord Lieutenant, General Martin White, was very involved with St John and, knowing of their official roles within St John, when he was organising visits by HRH the Duke of Gloucester to Osborne House and by the Countess of Wessex to Haseley Manor made sure that the visits involved meeting St John volunteers.

In London and in other parts of the country many of the non-sporting events are larger and often involve the provision of first aid for many thousands of people. Over the years amongst other events I was involved in covering several Armistice Day parades and the evening concerts that followed, Trooping the Colours and royal weddings. The majority of my work was at sporting events and with the Royal Protection Group. For seventeen years I was regularly on duty at Lords for the test matches, including one where there was a royal visit, at Wimbledon for the tennis championships, and at Twickenham for the rugby, which included World Cup matches, and I was also part of the medical team which covered two London marathons. As a doctor I was in a privileged position and normally was able to watch most of the competition. Over the years I did have to give medical care to a considerable number of patients, most of whom were spectators and not players. The luckiest person was a man queuing to get into Twickenham who had a heart attack and cardiac arrest. The person behind him in the queue as he collapsed was a doctor, and when we arrived, about two minutes later, he was already receiving CPR (cardio-pulmonary resuscitation). Oxygen and a defibrillator were attached, and when I pressed the button his heart restarted, and he rapidly recovered. He was sent into hospital where two stents were inserted into arteries supplying blood to his heart, and he went home to Wales, a new man, the next day. I am not sure that he realised how lucky he was to have had his heart attack where and when it happened.

The crowds watching rugby are totally different from soccer crowds. There is no separation of spectators supporting the opposing teams, and it is almost unheard of for there to be trouble between them. On one occasion, though, and no one did discover why, an American spectator was attacked at the end of the match and knocked unconscious. He rapidly recovered, but as a USAF pilot, having been rendered unconscious, he was not allowed to fly for a week. I would normally see the whole of the match as people would admit to being ill before or after the game, but rarely during it. On my last duty at Twickenham, however, I saw none of the match as two people had heart attacks during the game. Both were sent into hospital and survived. Before the match started on two occasions Richard Bunsell the anaesthetist from Stoke Mandeville came in to the first aid room to say hello. He was there as the resuscitation officer for the players during the match, and was working with Nigel Henderson, an orthopaedic surgeon and friend, also from Stoke Mandeville, who was covering injuries to the English team.

From 2002 until 2018 I was on duty at the Wimbledon tennis championships, and in most years I would do two days in each of the two weeks. With the exception of the London Marathon, that duty was far busier than any other that I did. There were four to six doctors on duty, and we covered three main first aid centres and one minor centre. We would work a half-hourly rotation, and normally have some time off. However, if the weather was very warm and the sun was out, we knew that there were going to be people collapsing, particularly on Court 1, where until the last few years no shade was provided. The secondary problem was that they could then fall down the concrete steps and do themselves more damage, occasionally quite severe.

One always remembers patients who were a little bit unusual. By far the worst was a retired American senator who collapsed in the gentlemen's lavatory. This was next door to the Centre Court first aid room and no time was lost before he was treated. Despite the best efforts of everybody, which included our senior consultant Dr Fenella Wrigley, we were unable to resuscitate him. We found out afterwards from his son, whom he had come to visit, that he had arrived on a plane that morning. From the history and examination, he had clearly suffered a deep vein thrombosis, where a blood clot had broken off from a vein in his leg and passed into his heart and lungs, causing the heart to stop.

I also remember a 14-year-old boy who on his way in had suddenly complained of a severe pain in his lower abdomen. Very reasonably, the first aiders had thought that this would be appendicitis. But when I examined him, there was a very obvious hernia in his right groin which had become strangulated. This caused the blood supply to be cut off, which caused the pain. I had seen this before in adults, but never in a child, and I later found out that it is extremely rare. The lad was very upset when I told him and his mother that he was off to the hospital, and no, despite his pleas, it could not wait until the end of play. Without an urgent operation, permanent damage would have occurred. I am delighted to say that Wimbledon gave him a free ticket for the following year.

The Centre Court first aid room also looked after the umpires, linesmen and the ball-boys and girls. I would normally be allocated to this room and the rule was that any of the former, whether serious or not, had to be checked by a doctor. In the first week the ball-boys and girls were rarely seen, but as the second week progressed various aches and pains developed. These were rarely serious.

Wimbledon was different from any other duty in that I was permitted to carry out minor surgery with a local anaesthetic. One day I remember doing three operations, one to remove a deeply embedded splinter, one to release pus from a deep ulcer, and the third to suture a facial laceration from a fall. That patient was very impressed to find that St John could provide a consultant plastic surgeon to do the operation! There were compensations. We were given a car park ticket and food, which was very generously provided. On occasions there was an additional Centre Court ticket for a wife/husband or friend, and the doctors were given one Centre Court ticket between us. Very occasionally we were too busy to use these! As we walked around the outer courts there was tennis to be seen, and I would make a special effort to see Mansour Bahrami in the senior men's doubles. He was quite brilliant, both as a tennis player and as an entertainer. In the first years when I was covering the No. 1 Court first aid centre, during quiet periods I could walk onto the area where players entered and stand there watching the play and seeing the players. This unfortunately was stopped for no obvious reason. When I finished work and handed in my medical licence in 2018, I was presented with a Certificate of Appreciation and presents from my colleagues and from Wimbledon.

As well as working for St John at headquarters organising the First Responders, John Newman was himself a keen cricketer and had taken on the responsibility of organising the first aid cover for the Marylebone Cricket Club at the Lords cricket ground. He had already recruited me when I was also working at HQ. From 2002 until 2018 I did two of the days for almost all home test matches at Lords. Although it had been enormously developed since my first visit as a young lad of 13 years old, nostalgia set in during my first return visit. I had been taken there in 1952 by a neighbour from home. In those days safeguarding had not been invented, and in that case was certainly not relevant. We had sat on the grass opposite the pavilion and I watched Peter May make 74 against India. Also in the English team were Hutton, Graveney and Truman.

The first aid facilities were far less good than at Wimbledon. In 2002 there was a small first aid room in the Warner stand, with two ambulances parked nearby, and a treatment ambulance on the other side of the ground behind the Edrich stand. The equipment was less and there were certainly no facilities for doing any surgery. After the rebuild of the Warner stand in 2016 there was a small improvement. The doctors and one ambulance crew had seats in front of the Warner stand, and the first aiders were either in the first aid facilities or on seats in the various stands. John Newman was in the control room with the senior policeman and the senior ambulance man, where via television they could see any problems and control the situation from there. The senior medic was normally Dr Tom Evans, a consultant cardiologist, and he would direct the most appropriate of the three doctors to any incident, or to the first aid room/ambulance. If Tom was not present on any day that I was there, the role was passed to me. The days were long and started with a briefing at 8.30am, and finished one and a half hours after the close of play. This could mean finishing at 8.30pm. Unfortunately there was free parking only at weekends, about half a mile away, and otherwise there could be a considerable wait for public transport.

In the first few years the doctors lunched in the players' dining room when they had finished. When in uniform under St John rules, we were not allowed to drink alcohol. The chief waiter, a marvellous Frenchman, would always ask in his French accent whether we wanted red or white water today. I will not elucidate further. In later years the doctors ate with all of the first aiders and the police in the indoor cricket pavilion, which was less interesting.

The five patients that I particularly remember had very different problems. The first was a man from the Royal Air Force, who was on crowd duty. He appeared with a very obvious but unusual rash. It was the first and only example of Lyme's disease that I have seen. It was so unusual, with what looked like small archery targets with a white centre, that I recognised it instantly. On questioning, he told me that he had just returned from manoeuvres in arctic Scandinavia, which confirmed the diagnosis.

The next patient came into the first aid room shivering on a warm day. He had had a urological operation two days before and had been fine on the morning that I saw him, and then suddenly became ill. He was clearly having an episode of severe sepsis. We had no antibiotics available, and I sent him into hospital as a blue light emergency, and phoned the hospital to warn them of the emergency. He received intravenous antibiotics and survived. I received a very nice letter afterwards.

The third patient was an elderly blind man who had tripped up on a pavement and fractured his femur. He was splinted, given analgesia and sent into hospital. I never did discover why a blind man was attending a cricket match.

The next patient was a man in his 80s who had fallen on the top floor of the new Warner stand. He was unconscious when we got to him, and he could have injured his neck as well as his head. I therefore put him in a neck collar, and we strapped him onto a stretcher. Unfortunately the person who had designed the new stand had not talked to anybody medical, and it was not possible to fit the stretcher into the lift. The alternative was to carry the patient on the stretcher down three levels of a spiral staircase. Clearly this would be difficult. Luckily some service personnel had been watching our first aid and suddenly found themselves with a job. Fit as they were, even they looked fairly exhausted when they had brought the patient down to the first aid room, where he recovered fully.

The final patient had been referred to us by the management. She had arrived by air with her famous retired cricketing husband that morning, but had been unwell on the flight and had been advised that she should be checked over on arrival in a hospital. I therefore took them both to St Mary's Hospital, and when I mentioned her name the speed with which she was seen was very impressive. Happily she checked out with no

Plastic Surgery in Wars, Disasters and Civilian Life

problem. I did not discover whether he had a large number of autographs to sign.

There were two personal remembrances. Firstly I fielded a ball in front of the pavilion! The television report must have been short that day, as my fielding appeared on national television that evening. The other occasion was the presentation of my St John long service award by the secretary of the MCC in front of the pavilion during my last match there.

Within St John in London there is a group of doctors, nurses, paramedics and first aiders known as the Designated Team. The members of this team are assessed at Operation Try-out at Bodney, and if selected then return for the three-day course every two or three years. The team works with the Royal Protection Group of the Metropolitan Police to provide first aid cover for the royal family and senior politicians on state occasions, and particularly if a procession of carriages is to take place. I was part of this team from 2002 until 2018. When I finished, I was presented with the tie, and told that I had been appointed an honorary member of the group. It is a tie that I now wear with pride.

Much of this work is for obvious reasons secret, and it must be a very difficult job for the police. They rehearse for a variety of possibilities, and very thankfully no member of the royal family has been injured since the assassination of Earl Mountbatten in 1979, and that was not on a state occasion. The last disaster was in 1982, when during the Changing of the Guards ceremony the IRA detonated a bomb that killed four guardsmen and eight horses.

I have much enjoyed the duties that I have done, which have included Armistice Day Parades, the State Opening of Parliament and the concert that follows in the evening at the Albert Hall, Trooping the Colour, the Chelsea Flower Show and the state visits of President Bush and the Norwegian royal family, and the unveiling of the memorial to Bomber Command in Piccadilly. My most regular events have been the Order of the Garter Parade and Service at Windsor Castle and a day or two at Royal Ascot. On one occasion I was standing by the door to the royal box in my morning suit and HRH the Duchess of Gloucester came up to me and said how nice it was to see me again. The only problem was that we had never met, but I managed to make a comment that passed muster. Another event that I covered many times was the Garden of Remembrance event at Westminster Abbey where ex-servicemen and family members place crosses, decorated with a name and a poppy, into the ground in their thousands. Except at Windsor and Ascot, the team rarely operates outside London, but I did cover the visit of Princess Anne to the 70th Anniversary of D-Day at Southsea. I have also been on duty at some military events both in the Palace and at Westminster Abbey. On one occasion the author and ex-serviceman George MacDonald Fraser was in the pulpit at the Abbey telling the story of when he and his colleagues had been released from a prisoner-of-war camp in the Far East. He suddenly, and unaccompanied, burst into song – the song that they had sung on the occasion sixty years earlier. He had a marvellous voice, and it was extremely moving.

Alternating with the Red Cross, we also covered Buckingham Palace garden parties. Annually there are four parties, at which those attending are recommended by the various Lords Lieutenant of all the counties. Her Majesty and several other members of the royal family attend these general parties. There are also special parties which vary yearly but may cover the Duke of Edinburgh's awards, centenaries of organisations such as the Boys Brigade, the Women's Institute and the Scouts. At one of these I very briefly met Boris Johnson. The very special party is the Not Forgotten Association party. This was originally to remember and to thank those who had fought in the Far East during the last war and who became known as the Forgotten Army. This party is smaller in numbers and now that the Forgotten Army members slowly fade away, also includes any serviceman who has been injured on duty. As invited guests there are well known people from the stage and television. One person whom I was very privileged to meet was Dame Vera Lynn. Because of the war service of St John this event is always ours, and because of the numbers present there is a much better chance to talk to people.

The garden parties can be quite busy medically, as most of the people attending are fairly old, but by far the commonest problems that we had to deal with were blisters. Ladies often wear new shoes without realising that soft grass is not ideal for them. One friend of mine, who regularly attends as part of the Diplomatic Corps, always arrives in old shoes which she then hands to me to look after in the medical centre as she puts on her new shoes. The Not Forgotten Party can cause many more problems, especially some years ago when the average age was much higher. There is also a very strong emotional effect on old soldiers meeting their colleagues of sixty years ago. At one party, whilst they were waiting to come in, three of them collapsed, and when in the gardens another three followed suit. Two had to go into hospital, even before they had entered the grounds. Happily, all of them survived.

The first garden party that I attended was with my wife, as an invited guest. In those days, and it has now changed, one could take unmarried daughters between the ages of 18 and 25. Both my daughters just fell within these limits and came with us. One is only normally allowed to attend one party but as I was also invited by HRH the Duke of Kent to the Jubilee Party and concert, I did not have to go as a St John volunteer. And when my wife was invited as the guest, somehow it was missed that we had both been before and we went again. With those three, and my duty attendances, I have now been to more than thirty parties. On two occasions I have very briefly met Her Majesty, and on another met HRH the Duke of Gloucester, who told me the following joke: 'You know that Prince Charles is very green – so why does he use petrol made from Welsh cheese?' 'So that he can drive Caerphilly!'

I still continue with St John. In 2013 the county structure was abolished, and the Ambulance part became national. Up to then we had a part-time secretary, Carol Young, who was also a volunteer. But we lost her and several other members, both volunteers and paid trainers. Our administration moved to the mainland, our numbers both of adults and of the cadets and badgers shrank very markedly, and to a large part through the efforts of Major Randal Cross we just about continued to exist. We lost most of the events on the island that we had previously covered, as these were taken over by professional first aiders, of whom several had been trained by St John. It was an unhappy time, and apart from the newly appointed managers, I know of no one who approved of this change.

The council within the county disappeared, and the Priory developed what were called County Priory Groups (CPGs). As many of the members were influential on the island, the role of these groups was to raise money and to keep alive the concept of St John. The other roles were to act as the body that recommended people for St John and other awards, and to organise joint presentations with the NHS to the families of people who had allowed organ donations from their deceased relatives. These latter we held at Haseley Manor, with either the Lord Lieutenant, General Martin White, or the High Sheriff of the year giving the medal and certificate to a family member. It was extremely moving for us all.

The CPG was by then completely divorced from the Ambulance branch. I was appointed chair of the CPG and moved my voluntary role to London, where the vast majority of my work had been. In 2019, after giving up my licence to practise, I was appointed as the president of St John Ambulance on the island. After considerable discussion nationally,

I was accredited as an Advanced First Aider, and after further arguments became both a trainer and assessor. I started teaching until early 2020, when the pandemic stopped all teaching.

One thing that St John has always done well is to recognise good and useful service, and also length of service. These are separate. The Priory makes appointments within the Order, and the Ambulance gives the awards for length of service. I was made a Member of the Order in 2013 and was promoted to Officer in 2019. I received my long-service award in 2013, and the first bar to this in 2018. The OBE that I had received was partly for services to the Isle of Wight, which included my work for St John.

St John has also given me the opportunity to continue my medical work at a lower level, which has been ideal as I have become older. There are frustrations. One has been that we very rarely discover what happens to our patients, particularly when they are admitted to hospital. And as I have found during my life, there are incompetent managers who think they are far more important than is the case.

Finally the pandemic has very much changed the duties of St John first aiders, who are now becoming vaccinators, as has my wife. Hopefully life will return to normal, and we can then try to increase the presence of St John both on the island and also nationally. Some good news is that several experienced Red Cross volunteers have now moved to St John. I am convinced that St John is an organisation that has shown enormous merit and much change – but certainly not all to the good.

Chapter 9

Overseas Teaching, Work and Conferences

Introduction

I have travelled widely throughout my life, both in Britain and overseas, and for various reasons. My travels began during the war with my father's postings, and then later I travelled for universities, work, natural history and for enjoyment. These will be described in fuller detail in another book.

My overseas travels started with the Scouts, and then accompanying my mother to visit friends who had moved overseas to Denmark and to Jersey. This was followed by travelling for sport, and then for education. I started travelling for medical teaching and for work overseas, to Zambia, and have continued travelling since. Some of these travels have been specifically for medical work, some for teaching, but in many, for instance my expeditions to fifteen countries, the medical role has been only a small part of the expedition. My role on these expeditions has been as medical officer, but thankfully my skills have been rarely needed.

On virtually all of my travels to the 107 countries that I have visited there has almost always been time available for natural history study or for normal tourism. I worked out in my early medical travels that setting aside a few days after the main purpose of the visit gave me an opportunity to meet people and to see places, often with the aid of help or introductions from colleagues that we had met at the conference or hospital in which I had lectured or operated. On many of my visits I was accompanied by Vivian, and also on occasions by one or both of my daughters.

Sweden

Stoke Mandeville Hospital was world famous for the first spinal injuries centre in the world. I knew from attending hand surgery conferences that enormous improvements in the function of quadriplegic patients could be gained by hand surgery. This particular type of surgery had been developed by Dr Eric Moberg in Gothenburg, Sweden. In 1986 I therefore organised a two-week attachment to his unit to learn the various operations, their successes and their complications. I was made extremely welcome by Eric, who was almost retired from active surgery, but was very much present in the department. His surgical successor was Dr Arvid Ejeskar, who took me under his wing. I assisted at a variety of operations and also learned about the physiotherapy and occupational therapy which followed.

I had one slightly embarrassing moment. During the two weeks there had been organised a two-day Scandinavian hand surgery conference. In his opening speech, Eric announced that there were overseas visitors, one from England and two from France. The papers would therefore be presented in English. I felt sorry for the Scandinavian presenters, but they managed unbelievably well. Unfortunately, the two Frenchmen did less well, and with my extremely outdated French I had to translate for them.

When I returned home, I had long conversations with two of the older spinal injury consultants but could not prove to them the value to their patients of the surgery. Looking back, I think perhaps that this failure was due to the fact that I had only just started working at Stoke, and they did not know me. Had two or three patients been successful, then they would have talked to each other, and I would have been very busy.

Nevertheless, the techniques I learnt were very useful in Sarajevo with the patients with war-damaged arm and hand nerves.

Overseas Professorships, Lectureships and Conferences as a Consultant

Conferences

In any hospital there are regular meetings and discussions about changes that have happened, about research and about problems that may have arisen in that hospital. There are similar meetings at both a national and an international level, and it is of major importance that practising doctors attend these as improvements and problems can be communicated both more rapidly and more accurately. It can be argued that the research is published in journals and can be read there, but this may often take many years. Also in a meeting, and in the social time before and afterwards, if one had been interested in a paper then the presenter can be questioned, and this is not possible when a paper is published in a journal.

Overseas Teaching, Work and Conferences

An example of the importance of this of which I have knowledge was the introduction of early surgery for burns. Mr Douglas Jackson was working at the Birmingham Accident Hospital when he heard a paper given by a Czech surgeon at a meeting in Eastern Europe, was impressed, and having found further details, introduced the method to Britain almost certainly several years earlier than it would otherwise have happened. It was a revolution in the treatment of many burn patients (*see* Chapter 2). Likewise, Mr Tom Barclay, working in Bradford, heard in the United States a paper on tissue expansion of skin. We did much of the British work when I was training in Yorkshire, and it again showed the advantages to treatment. Both of these are now standard treatment methods throughout this and other countries.

I have regularly attended meetings in burn care, hand surgery and general plastic surgery both annually in Britain and also internationally to keep up to date with new methods around the world.

The meetings to which I have been invited in countries such as Bosnia and Kosovo, just emerging from war, have I think given them encouragement, and given me the opportunity to see where aid would be helpful, and this I have on occasions been able to support by arranging visits both ways.

Conferences also have other uses, one of which is the opportunity for doctors, and particularly doctors in training, to present their research. These papers are noted in their CVs and if they have been well received, can aid their selection for promotion.

A third use that I have found in my retirement is remaining friends with old colleagues. I still go to (or did before Covid) military conferences, including those of the Military Surgical Society and the Combined Services Plastic Surgery Society, to meet my old trainees and colleagues. It is also of interest to discover any recent changes. There are always stories arising at such conferences. A favourite of mine occurred in Hong Kong, where apparently travelling Americans could only claim their expenses against tax if they presented a paper. This need does mean that those presentations may be of a rather poor content. The paper that I remember was a new method being presented of which the surgeon had done just one case. After the presentation, when questions were requested, a Chinese surgeon said, 'I have done more than fifty of these operations, and you are talking rubbish.' Some gentle chuckles ensued, but it was difficult not to roar with laughter.

Australia
My first overseas conference was the International Society for Burn Injuries Conference in Melbourne in 1986 where I presented a paper on the Bradford Fire, which aroused considerable interest and discussion.

In 1993 I was awarded the Travelling Professorship of the International Society of Burn Injuries. My first task was to visit the University of Western Australia in Perth, where I presented my work on the early surgery of burns. I also had long discussions with Dr Fiona Wood about her development of spray-on skin, which is now a standard treatment.

South Africa
I was asked at the 1986 conference in Australia if I would present the same work at the Plastic and Reconstructive Surgeons of Southern Africa Conference in 1987. This developed into a three-week visit, funded by a pharmaceutical company, which with the Association had arranged an extremely busy tour for me. I presented the Bradford Fire experience at six universities in South Africa with a medical school, and these lectures were followed by presenting six papers at the Association Conference at the Sani Pass Conference Centre. This included a national radio broadcast on the equivalent of the BBC's 'Today' programme (see below). At the end of my visit I was elected an Honorary Member of the Association and have since returned to their conferences in the Kruger National Park and in Stellenbosch. At the former I gave one paper.

In 2017, whilst visiting my daughter in Cape Town, I made contact with an old colleague, Professor Hans Rode. He asked me to visit the Red Cross Children's Hospital and give a paper on the treatment of paediatric burns.

Hong Kong and China
In 1989, completely out of the blue, came an invitation from Ms Alison Liu of the legal part of the government there to fly to Hong Kong to examine and report on the severe contractures of three young men who had been burned in an industrial accident. I flew out and was met by three lawyers and then introduced to the patients. They indeed had severe contractures of their limbs of such severity that they would not be able to do a manual job. I discussed through the lawyers what was possible, and it was suggested that they be flown to England for treatment. One problem with this was that the three patients spoke no English, and this would have made the nursing care very difficult. Instead I suggested that we could look into the possibility of me returning to Hong Kong to do the

Overseas Teaching, Work and Conferences

operations there. Very surprisingly, at that time there was no plastic surgery within the Chinese University of Hong Kong. However, there was a very good department of surgery under Professor Arthur Li, and Dr Walter King, one of the senior staff, had an interest in reconstruction. He readily agreed that I would be able to do the operations at the Prince of Wales Hospital in Sha Tin, and arrangements were made for me to return later that year. I was also requested to do some teaching during the coming visit. There was an interesting situation in plastic surgery in Hong Kong at that time, as once a plastic surgeon had been trained, they immediately went full-time private, leaving no suitable expertise available for the university hospitals. When I returned I was able to stay with long-term friends Tony and Jan Galsworthy. He was a China expert and had been posted by the Foreign Office to be in charge of the negotiations for the return of Hong Kong to China in 1997. When he heard that I was to give a lecture, his comment was that no one would laugh at my jokes, and the professor only would ask two questions. I was extremely grateful for the warning, as that was exactly what happened. The surgery was reasonably successful, and I was invited to return whenever I could, and even more importantly the university would fund my travel and look after me. This suited me extremely well as Tony was a fellow bird-ringer. My future visits were therefore planned to coincide with the timing of the bird migration, which had the secondary advantage that I did not have to suffer the very hot and humid summers or the relatively cold winters.

I organised the future visits by flying out on the Friday, arriving at 4.00pm and then visiting the patients in the hospital. Then it was straight to bed and up in the early hours on the Saturday to go bird-ringing. By Monday morning, when Walter would collect me from Tony and Jan's house near the peak on Hong Kong Island, my jet lag had disappeared and I was ready to operate. One or two weeks later I would fly home on the Sunday, with take-off at dusk, and arriving at Heathrow as dawn was breaking, to be in the operating theatre at Stoke Mandeville by 9.00am. I have never discovered why jet lag is so much less when flying east, but it certainly is.

Work during these visits involved both operating and lecturing to junior staff or at the international surgical conferences that were regularly organised. There was one particularly interesting invitation which was on the foundation of the Hong Kong Burn Association in 1993. I was asked to talk about how, on a national scale, burn injuries were managed in the United Kingdom. Dr David Herndon from the United States was to talk about the management in the USA. During my lecture he made copious notes and he worked out from our comparative figures that burn deaths were twice as common per head of population in the United States compared to Britain. When discussing this afterwards, we found that the real difference was in death rates in industrial accidents. In Britain we often moan about the Health and Safety Executive and its rules, but it became clear to me then that we should stop moaning and thank them for their success.

In 1996 I was appointed to the prestigious C C Wu Professorship in the Department of Surgery and visited the university to give my appointment lecture, as well as several other teaching sessions. One of these was to the trainee surgeons and senior medical students. By this time they were used to my lectures, which had become easier on both sides. The Chinese are very wary of laughing at a joke during a lecture or conversation in case it is thought that they are laughing at the lecturer and not the joke. The other thing about Chinese humour is that it is very basic and earthy. I had been talking about burns, where one of the problems encountered can be severe diarrhoea. One of the audience asked what could be done for this. I replied that the best treatment was to buy a bottle of champagne, drink the fizz and use the cork in the patient. It was the only time that laughter echoed round the lecture theatre.

About two years later Walter had moved more and more towards plastic surgery and a professorship had been created, for which he applied. He asked me to be his referee. When I saw the terms of the post, I nearly tore up the reference that I had written for him and applied myself.

I had had two earlier short trips combined with the Hong Kong visits, one to China and one to Thailand, and both were with Vivian. The first involved a coach trip into Guangdong Province, where we visited Guangzhou, and then drove halfway to Guilin and visited the home of Dr Sun Yat Sen, the first President of the new Chinese Republic. The second visit, some years later, was to Chang Mai in Thailand, close to the Burmese border. My main memory there was a very uncomfortable ride on an elephant. Without the work in Hong Kong, these trips would not have occurred when they did.

I was invited to the handover of Hong Kong to China in 1997 but could not free up the time needed. I only returned to Hong Kong once afterwards, in 1998. Having lectured there, I flew from Hong Kong with Mr Alan Collins, the British Ambassador to the Philippines, who had been visiting Hong Kong, to Beijing, and very much enjoyed being taken through the diplomatic channel at the airport, missing the enormous queues. We were staying with our old friends Tony and Jan Galsworthy; Tony was by then the British Ambassador in Beijing, and he had organised for me to visit and to lecture in three university hospitals. The first was the 304th Military Hospital, which was an excellent centre, where I lectured in English on research in burns. During my visit I was introduced to the retired director of the hospital, aged 91. As I left, the present director confided in me that the past director insisted on visiting the hospital every day and kept telling him what to do. This was obviously very difficult as there is an enormous respect for age in China. The second lecture was to the First Teaching Hospital of the University of Peking on burn treatment, and the third was to the Peking University Medical College on new developments in burn treatment. Both of these were given with consecutive translation. This makes lecturing more difficult and takes much longer. One also wonders what is being translated when a joke has been cracked and there is no response, and then the next sentence without a joke, causes laughter.

I was invited to return to China in July 2013 to teach at a Disaster Conference, which at the request of the Chinese had been organised in Chengdu in western China, an are where earthquakes were common. There had been a disastrous one in 2008 in Wenchuan, close to Chengdu, when nearly 70,000 people died and a further 316,000 were injured. The course was along the lines of the ATLS courses, but as China was not registered with the American College of Surgeons, none of that material could be used. I am delighted to say that this time simultaneous translation was used. Even this can cause problems. I had been explaining why the degrees of burn depth were no longer used, but, according to the Chinese speaker in our group, the translator was still using the old terms. She rapidly corrected him. Sichuan Province in the far west was very different from Hong Kong. The food was incredibly spicy and alcohol was drunk in large quantities. The outstanding visit on this trip was to the panda reserve.

When I was retiring from the NHS, Walter King suggested that I join him to work privately in Hong Kong as a plastic and hand surgeon. He said that in working three months of the year there I would earn more than I was earning with my combined NHS and private work in England. However, we had just bought our new manor, so I decided to turn down the very kind and tempting offer.

India

I had arranged to present the Bradford Fire experience at the International Society for Burn Injuries Conference in Delhi in 1991. Burn injuries are a very common cause of death in India. Mr Douglas Jackson, after his retirement from Birmingham, had visited India on behalf of the World Health Organization and had estimated that around 100,000 people a year died there from burns. Perhaps because of this, six of the more experienced delegates from around the world were asked to go to a different centre each in India for a week to teach after the conference. We were given a special and almost private visit to the Taj Mahal, and I, accompanied by Vivian, was then sent to Ahmedabad, the capital city of Gujerat. Dr P.K. Bilwani, to whom I had been introduced at the conference, was the person in charge of the large burn unit at the BJ Medical College Hospital. I did a long ward-round and in the discussion at the end I was asked what I thought were the most important things on which they needed to spend money, as no burned patient with more than 20 per cent burns had ever survived. I discovered that this figure also included children and was therefore a very poor survival rate indeed. With considerable efforts to remain polite, I tried to get across the fact that what was most needed was that the place needed cleaning, and the staff needed to wash their hands and wear the correct sterile gloves and dress, which must be changed between each patient.

The next part of the conversation began with 'Which ones do you want to operate on tomorrow?' I pointed out that I was not registered in India, but the reply came, 'Oh we do not worry about that.' And so I operated very full-time for the next two days. I must have been sufficiently polite as I was asked to return to Ahmedabad several times.

During one visit I was extremely surprised to receive an invitation to dine with the Governor of the Gujarat. At the end of the excellent dinner (minimally spoiled as Gujarat is a dry state), the reason for the invitation became clear. He had a surgical son who wanted a training appointment in England. I had to point out how the system in the UK worked, which was very different from India, and that although he was welcome to come as a visitor, he would have to undergo a competitive interview for an official appointment. I heard no more.

The other contact that I had there was Dr Sanjiv Vasa. We had worked together as junior doctors in Leeds, and in 1991 he was working privately in Ahmedabad. I was able to see his work, and my wife and I stayed with Sanjiv and Purnima on three visits. On one of my visits I was asked by

Overseas Teaching, Work and Conferences

Professor Malti Gupta if, together with a German hand surgeon, we would organise the first Indian microsurgical course. We duly organised a four-day course in Jaipur in 1993 at which twelve doctors attended. It was an interesting challenge. We asked to be supplied with live rats for demonstrations and for the candidates to use for practice. Unfortunately we did not specify the ideal size of the rats, and those provided were little bigger than mice. It was a surgical challenge. The second part of the course was dissecting cadavers to show simple vascular flaps. This was much easier than in Europe, as there were ample cadavers made available, apparently those of homeless and family-less people who had died.

Whilst I was there, a Dalit student had self-immolated as a protest and was brought into the burn unit by fifty or sixty of his university colleagues. They demanded that Malti save him, but she knew his burns were unsurvivable. This was obviously an extremely dangerous situation but Malti solved it quite brilliantly. She told all of the students that they each needed to donate a pint of blood. Giving blood, except in desperation for relatives, was not common in India, and except for three students the unit emptied very rapidly.

Jaipur, the pink city, was a stunning place. There was a welcoming meeting presided over by the dowager Maharana of Jaipur, who was a delightful older lady. Vivian and I stayed with Anil and Mona Maheshwaray, who were relatives of Malti. Over the week we became friendly and conversations broadened. During one discussion about corruption in India I asked if, giving enough cash to the appropriate person, Anil could commit murder. He thought about it for a minute – and said almost certainly.

My final visit to India was in 1999 at the invitation of one of my old trainees to give the second Kannapan Shanmuganathan Oration at the Ganga Hospital in Coimbatore in the State of Tamil Nadu in the south of India. This hospital, now world famous, has an almost unbelievable story. Raja Sabapathy was an outstanding plastic surgery trainee who came to England with his orthopaedic trainee brother Dr Rajasekeran in 1987 or 1988. Raja spent eighteen months with our unit at Stoke Mandeville. When he had been with us for about six months, he asked if he could have a day of leave, which was considerably overdue. When he came into the hospital the day after his leave, he was asked what he had done on his day off. 'I passed the Fellowship of the College,' he said. We did not even know that he had been working for it. From us, he moved to the unit in Glasgow, and then he, his brother and their wives returned to India.

There they took over their father's private six-bed hospital and began to develop it as a trauma centre with Raja as the plastic surgeon, his wife as the manager, his brother as the orthopaedic surgeon and his wife as the matron, and their father as the anaesthetist. It was still a private hospital, run on marvellous Hindu lines, where people were charged what they could afford – which might be nothing. Further finance came from local companies and from generous donors, and after one of them was named the Oration that I gave. With another of my hats on, the son of this person was also a Formula 1 driver for a time. When I was there the hospital had grown to hold more than one hundred beds and now, in 2020, there are several hundred beds and it is world famous, with a long waiting list of trainees wanting to go there to study as Fellows. One of the Fellowships is named after my old senior colleague, the late Bruce Bailey. That visit had been combined with a meeting of the Indian Plastic Surgeons in Madras, and then travelling down via Bangalore.

I valued my multiple visits to India. The medical service was completely different from that in the United Kingdom. There was a state system, but with exceptions at a low or very low level. The majority of health care was in small private facilities where money was very important. And then there were outstanding places such as the Ganga Hospital.

Israel
I attended a burn conference in Israel in 1992. Many of the papers concerned tank warfare and the resulting burns. Most interesting was a visit to Hadassah Hospital to see a mock disaster practice. This was much better than the practices that I had been involved with in England, and I was able to institute some changes for the next one that we did at Stoke Mandeville.

United States of America
In 1992 I was on a family holiday in the United States. Having a day to spare, I contacted the burn unit at the University of California in Los Angeles. It was an interesting experience as the director was also the Professor of Medical Ethics. Burn care in the United States was based on the same system as in Australia. Burn surgery there is a specialty of general surgery, and not of plastic surgery as it is in the UK and most of Europe. This makes a difference to reconstruction work, particularly for children, as the patients are transferred between specialties for reconstructive work.

In 1998 I presented a paper at the International Societies of Hand Surgeons in Vancouver, Canada, and afterwards we drove south to Seattle, where I visited Dr David Heimbach at the Harbourview Hospital. This was a very interesting visit. At the time David was President of the International Society for Burn Injuries and he had presented his work at the hospital at various meetings. I was therefore surprised to find that the unit was smaller than mine at Stoke Mandeville, and had less patient throughput in a year. I was, however, very envious of the research grants that he was getting from the Boeing Aircraft Company in the town.

Papua New Guinea
For the second part of my Professorship of the International Society for Burn Injuries I flew from Western Australia to Port Moresby in Papua New Guinea and spent a very full week there teaching and lecturing at their Annual Medical Conference. It was an unusual event for me as I was lecturing to doctors of all subjects and of all levels. Port Moresby was an unsafe city, and we were accompanied by an armed guard at all times and were strongly advised not to leave the hotel grounds in the dark. I was very much hoping for some time off to see some of the island's famous natural history, but only managed one afternoon in the grounds of the university.

Japan
I attended a hand surgery conference in Japan in 1995. This was the first visit for Vivian, Clare and me and we were expecting crowds everywhere – and perhaps especially on the trains. Amazingly the train from the airport to Tokyo centre had some policemen aboard, and almost nobody else. We discovered later that the dreadful Sarin poison attack on a train had occurred whilst we were in the plane. It made the first week somewhat worrying, as there was another potential attack whilst we were in Yokohama. There was an interesting conference, but regrettably I did not visit any hospitals. Afterwards we toured parts of Japan and visited Hakodate in the north, which was where Vivian's grandfather had set up his Bishopric as the first Bishop of North Japan.

Egypt
The Egyptian Army had an interesting method of training their doctors, and for keeping them up to date. In about 1990 I was asked to have, as a visitor, Dr Ezeldin Eldolify (known as Ez), who was a plastic surgical trainee who had been selected for a three-year training appointment in the UK. He was with us at Stoke Mandeville for about two months and was clearly exceptional. Unfortunately we did not have a vacancy coming up for a suitable post, and with my strong backing Ez therefore applied to other units, and was appointed elsewhere.

Plastic Surgery in Wars, Disasters and Civilian Life

The second half of their training system was for each specialty to invite two overseas consultants to Egypt each year, with their other halves, to operate and to teach for two weeks, and in payment they were then given a visit for three or four days anywhere in Egypt. I was honoured and delighted to be invited by Ez in 1997 for my first visit on this scheme.

I had previously visited Cairo on my way home from Zambia in 1969 and again in 1984 for a hand surgery joint meeting, where I presented a paper and then enormously enjoyed a cruise on the Nile with the delegates. Our visit in 1997 was very different. Vivian and I were flown out first class by Egyptair, and were treated as VIPs on arrival. Getting off the plane, we were met at the steps by a car, and then problems of passports and luggage were all organised as we sat drinking orange juice in the VIP lounge with a junior surgeon who had been deputed to meet us. This was definitely the way to travel! On the way to the hotel we had two minor scrapes in the unbelievable traffic. I complained about this the next day, and it turned out that the only licence the driver had was for motor-cycles. He did not drive us again. We were accommodated at the Sheraton Hotel on El Gezira island, and the next day, with Ez, visited the enormous Maadi Military Hospital as an introduction. I did some lecturing there, but as the major plastic surgery and burn unit was at the Helmia Military Hospital to the north, I spent the remainder of my time there doing clinics, operating and teaching.

This large and busy hospital to the north of Cairo treated military, ex-military and civilian patients. It included a 70-bed burn unit for both adults and children, which was far larger than any burn unit in Europe. The Director of the hospital was General Mohammed El-Sawy. On the wall in his office was a photograph of the famous English orthopaedic surgeon Professor James Charnley, who was to a large extent responsible internationally for hip replacement surgery. On questioning, I discovered that he had commanded the hospital for the British army during the Second World War.

My work there, and over the following eight visits, was a mixture of lecturing, teaching in out-patient clinics and operative teaching. There were many interesting occasions. One duty which became routine was to examine senior members of the Egyptian services and their children. Why they had to be seen by the overseas doctors when there were very adequate local doctors I never did discover. One very successful case was a general who was losing sensation and function in his right hand, and had a tender swelling just below his elbow. When we operated, it turned out to be a lipoma – a lump of fat – which was pressing on his median nerve. It was an excellent outcome, and Ez could easily have done the operation, but at least the reputation of British doctors was promoted. Another case was the wife of a general who wanted a face-lift. I told her that I had never done one, and did not really want to practise on her – to which she only reluctantly agreed as she was desperate for the operation. I did a hypospadias operation on the child of a military doctor. We had agreed that he would stay in the ward for a week whilst the swelling went down and he could be nursed without nappies. But he was taken home the following day, and I never did discover the outcome. Several of the children on the burn unit had been burned with phosphorus by the Israelis in Gaza, and had been brought to the Helmia with horrific burns. This had only recently happened and some early surgery was possible.

There were amusing times. I discovered early on that operating lists, and anything else except for prayers, never started on time. I therefore invented 'English Time'. When anything was organised, we would agree whether it started on English or Egyptian time. On my last visit I was due to meet Mrs Mubarak, the wife of the President. I had been well briefed as to what was needed by the hospital and for which I was to plead. For some reason the arrangement went wrong, and her visit was cancelled.

The other work and teaching that I did on two of my visits was at the medical school of the University of Zag-a-Zig, situated in the Nile estuary. This was through a contact of Ez, Professor Sobhi Hweidi. I gave a lecture on each of the visits and on one occasion I was asked to present the diplomas to the successful candidates on the excellent microsurgical course that Sobhi ran. This time I was somewhat successful in promoting the course on my return home, and some English trainees did later attend the course.

The social life on these visits was excellent. Firstly I was able to have somebody with me. Vivian came on three occasions, and our daughters came once each. During the working days there were meals, either in an officers' mess or on a river cruise. We visited the pyramids and all the local sights, including the Faiyum Oasis. And then, at the end we would go for three or four days to somewhere else in Egypt. I did three Nile cruises, went to Alexandria and to El Alamein, made two visits to Sharm el Sheikh and St Catherine's Monastery and another to Hurghada, and finally journeyed to Siwa Oasis close to the Libyan border.

I also had long fascinating discussions with Ez about Egyptian life and religion, and an excellent visit to Sobhi Hweidi's beautiful house for dinner. I bought some superb Egyptian artwork and had made some reproduction French furniture, which was common in Egypt. I hope that I contributed as much as I gained.

Russia

In 1997 I was invited to attend the First Russian-American Meeting on Burns and Fire Disasters. How it happened I am not sure, but I was the only non-American overseas attendee. The main conference was in St Petersburg, where Vivian and I spent two days staying with a Russian lady and her daughter in her house. As well as presentations at the conference, we also visited hospitals and saw the incredible sights of the city. The hospitals were fascinating. My assessment was that medicine in Russia was clearly on two levels. The lower level was relatively basic, and even the level of doctoring was below the standard of nursing in Britain. Looking at the achievements and research output, there was clearly a higher level as well – perhaps in the universities in the major cities. The conference then moved en-bloc to Moscow, where a further hospital visit was arranged, but no further presentations. Vivian and I then took trains to visit Latvia, Lithuania and Estonia on our way home – but were not involved in any of their medical systems.

Botswana

The year 1998 was a very full one for me in terms of overseas work. It started with a visit to Botswana, as I had suggested that Stoke Mandeville might be able to help with the plastic surgical work there. This followed other British units which were involved in helping West Africa. I had a very positive reply from Dr Howard Moffat, the senior doctor in the country, welcoming the idea of a visit, and even better he had arranged through the local High Commissioner, Mr John Wilde, that the FCO would pay for my fares and accommodation. Howard is an interesting man. He is both an ordained Christian minister and was also the President's personal physician. The wife of Dr Livingstone was a member of his family. I therefore arranged two weeks of leave and flew out. Interestingly I was in the back end of the plane. In the front end were British soccer referees on their way to teach in Botswana. Clearly soccer was more important than surgery!

Botswana is an interesting country. When my wife and I first visited it in 1974, it was one of the poorest countries in Africa. Then diamonds were discovered in enormous quantities, and by 1998 it was one of the richest countries, and also had one of the lowest rates of corruption. Less fortunately, it also had the highest measured rate of HIV infection in the world. But it is important that the word 'measured' is in that sentence as the government was very active, and in the capital, Gabarone, there was a large research laboratory working with Harvard University which had been established in 1996, and treatment was widely available. There was also a university which had a medical school. However, very few students were applying to read medicine. It turned out that a doctor qualifying from the university had to work for three years for the government at a low salary, and therefore the good students were applying to read law and computing which had no such tie, and they could make a lot more money.

On this visit I spent the whole of the two weeks in the Princess Marina Hospital in Gabarone, both teaching and operating. Also retired and working privately in Gabarone was a Scottish plastic surgeon, Dr Alastair Lamont, whom I had met as a consultant at Stellenbosch University in South Africa and who was helping on occasions. One of the local general surgeons had developed an interest in cleft lip and palate surgery, with good results. Burn injuries are very common in much of Africa and much of my teaching and work there was on burns and their treatment. I had one embarrassing moment. Thinking that technology might be a little behind in Botswana, I had taken my lectures on old-fashioned 35mm slides. When I got there they had considerable trouble in finding a suitable projector and were very much into discs. As was happening more and more, I also became somewhat involved in local politics. A surgeon had been working privately and there was considerable disquiet locally about some of his results. I was therefore asked to review some of the patients and write a report. This I did, and I understand that his licence was subsequently revoked. I also met the Minister of Health. We discussed amongst other things the problem of the medical school. I clearly failed to make the point about the three-year tie-in and the salary. I also pointed out that there was no satisfactory training scheme for young doctors progressing through the ranks. I was unimpressed with the minister, Mr C.J. Butale, and I understand that he left the post soon afterwards.

The hospital, the doctors and the nursing care were of an excellent standard compared to others in Africa in which I had worked. But the number of patients in the wards dying of AIDS was dispiriting. When operating we were all very careful, wearing double gloves and taking great care of all sharp objects.

I returned to Botswana in 2001 with Vivian and this time we stayed in the Moffat's cottage. The visit was more organised, as it incorporated a local conference in Francistown, as well as teaching and operating in Gabarone. I met with the new Minister of Health and was very impressed with her knowledge and with the programme that she was planning to introduce. We also met Dr Merriweather and his wife. We had arranged to meet him and visit his Scottish Mission Hospital in Molepolole in 1974. A fascinating man with an incredible history of service to Botswana, he had been the Health Minister as well as director of the hospital. We revisited that hospital, and also another Scandinavian Mission hospital. There I was asked to see a lady with severe contraction of one hand. It was a classic case of Dupuytren's Disease – which is extremely rare in Africans, with only a few hundred cases reported worldwide, mostly in black Americans. On close questioning she was sure that she had no European ancestors, but had suffered a serious injury to that hand some years previously. This is not uncommon in Dupuytren's cases. I operated on the hand and obtained a reasonable range of movement of the involved fingers.

In 2002 I returned for my last visit. Again I was teaching and operating. On this occasion I brought with me a letter from HRH the Duke of Kent to the hospital which had been named after his mother.

Azerbaijan
In the summers of 1998, 1999 and 2000 I visited the post-war zone in Azerbaijan for two weeks (*see* Chapter 6).

Spain
In the autumn of 1998 Professor McGrouther had been invited to present at a European meeting in Madrid. This proved impossible, and he asked me to go there in his stead and to present the work on disasters.

United Arab Emirates
In December 1998 I was asked by the Glasgow College of Surgeons to join a team of examiners in Abu Dhabi in the United Arab Emirates. On entry, we all had to declare ourselves as alcoholics, and then we could then be served alcohol in the hotel. The examination itself was in the main hospital, and I noticed on the way in a large building labelled Drug Addiction Centre. On questioning, this was mainly used for alcoholics, but luckily we were not admitted. The people being examined were both local and from India and Pakistan, as well as a smaller number from other countries. I did have several conversations and a visit to the clinic of an Egyptian paediatric surgeon who had been working there for several

years. He had recorded a large percentage of cases of rare congenital abnormalities, which he attributed to a high rate of inter-family marriage.

Philippines

In 1999 I was invited by the British Ambassador, Mr Alan Collins (later Sir Alan Collins), whom I had met the previous year in China, to visit the Philippines. There was a major problem there of burns from fireworks occurring at the time of one of their festivals, and he had some money from the FCO to try to prevent this, and to give advice on the treatment when an injury occurred. I stayed in the ambassador's house and did three programmes on their national television, which included one half-hour interview, and also various teaching sessions in three universities. The ambassador's wife Ann also persuaded me to give a talk about surgery to 10-year-old pupils at the International School in Manila. This was a first for me, and definitely the last! There were questions afterwards, and the first question, from an American boy, was, 'Gee, doc – how many times have you been sued?' I am certain that he did not believe me when I said that I had never been sued.

Vivian and I then flew to the island of Cebu, to teach in the University there and to operate in the hospital. We stayed with the British Consul, Mrs Moya Jackson, whose family ran a company making elegant reproduction furniture, and were introduced by her to the university and to the press.

My return visit to the Philippines for the typhoon disaster in 2013 is described in Chapter 6.

Romania

I attended a meeting concerned with charities working overseas in the Durbar Room of the Foreign and Commonwealth Office building in London in 2003 and discussed the possibility of me doing further work overseas with various other delegates. Out of this came an invitation for my wife and me from Patrick and Frances Colquhoun in Cambridge to join a visit by the charity Medical Support Romania in 2004. The charity had been donating money to the medical services and the hospital in Zalau in the north of the country. We were asked to go to help in the assessment of whether the money was being well spent, and to try to reduce corruption. We flew in via Hungary, and were then taken to the house of a local surgeon, Dr Dorel Dindelegan, where we stayed for the week. I did some teaching and one hypospadias operation with a local surgeon. We all knew that there was corruption – or at least paybacks to the doctors – as it would have been impossible for them to live in the houses, and own the cars, that they did on the government salaries, which were minimal. It was not obvious, with the exception of one anaesthetist who apparently had been telling his patients before putting them to sleep that unless he was paid extra they would not wake up! After our report, he was disbarred from practice. At the end of the week Dr Dindelegan had organised through his son George, also a surgeon, for me to lecture at the university in Kluj-Napoca, the second city in Romania. We had an interesting car journey south through Transylvania and there I met Professor Constantin Ciuce. He showed me round their microsurgical facility before I lectured on the surgery of burns in a magnificent old-style tiered lecture theatre, unfortunately with consecutive translation. On returning home I tried to promote their excellent microsurgical course to surgeons in England, but without success.

Bangladesh

At a British Plastic Surgeons conference I talked to Mr Ronald Hiles OBE, a retired consultant from Bristol who had been working as a visiting surgeon with the Acid Survivors Foundation in Bangladesh for several years. He suggested that I join him on a visit the following year, and in 2005 I did so. It is quite horrific that there is the need for a hospital in Dhaka which only treats burns caused by people pouring acid onto other people. These cases happen either because marriage has been refused or because of land disputes. The majority of the patients were young women, and mostly had facial burns. Approximately half were also blinded by the acid. The hospital was founded in 1999 by the Acid Survivors Foundation and is funded by them. The plastic surgery required was the same as is done for facial scarring, particularly from burns, and involved eyelid reconstruction in some of the patients. The hospital also acted as both an out-patient facility and as a meeting place for the discharged patients, who were often rejected by their families and by wider society.

Through one of the trainees working in the Acid Survivors Hospital I was introduced to the Dhaka University Hospital. There was there a large burn unit, where I both lectured and operated. There was a very different causation of the burns here from anywhere else in the world that I had worked. Nearly a third were from high voltage electricity, and often required amputations. Unbelievably many of these were workers from the electricity supply company, which had not isolated the part of the grid on which they had been working. Others had been stealing the electricity from overhead cables. At the end of my time I was made an honorary professor, and much regret that I have not had the chance to revisit the country. I did present the work at the British Burn Association Conference in Dublin the following year.

Cambodia

My wife and I visited Cambodia with friends in 2008. Our friends' daughter was working in Phnom Penh as a doctor and she suggested that I visited the Children's Surgical Centre. I was welcomed by Dr Jim Gologoly, a Yorkshireman and an orthopaedic surgeon, who on his retirement from the NHS had set up and was still directing the hospital. And, surprise, surprise, for the next day and a half I was operating on a badly burned child and her mother. The mother unfortunately died from her injuries some days later, but the child did survive.

Gibraltar

In 2014 my wife and I attended the British Military Surgical Society meeting in Gibraltar where I gave a paper on my experience following the Philippines typhoon. It is always interesting talking with military surgeons who have often had similar experiences.

Expeditions

I have been the appointed medical officer on British Schools Exploring Society (later the British Exploring Society) expeditions to Arctic Lapland, Peru and Iceland. On all these expeditions foot blisters were a common problem, but none became infected. I carried out an inconclusive trial of Micropore against Mepore for the better treatment/prevention of the blisters. On the Lapland expedition in 1976 there was often poor communication, and only the possibility of a helicopter rescue. The Birmingham Accident Hospital and several pharmaceutical companies were extremely helpful in providing instruments and medication, and I borrowed enough surgical equipment for fixing fractures and also for being able to do an appendicectomy if it had been necessary. In Lapland there was one case of hypothermia following a canoe accident, but the lad recovered without problems. There was also one case of a minor burn, when somebody broke the rules and used a gas stove in a small tent.

In Peru in 2006 I was asked by the young doctor on the expedition to look at a lad of 17 who had a thrombosed haemorrhoid. This is very rare in young people, but is often extremely painful. It is one of those conditions for which a minor and simple operation gives instant relief, and there are very few of those! I did this for him and he finished the expedition with no problems. The other issue on that expedition was that our base camp was at 3,200m (10,500ft), and we were working up to more than 4,000m (more than 13,000ft). Despite proper conditioning for that altitude, three people on the expedition became ill with altitude sickness. Two of these were leaders, and had mild symptoms, but the third was a 17-year-old boy who had more severe symptoms. All three had to be sent down to the base camp to recover. The very sad aspect of this for the young lad was that he was extremely fit and wanted to join the Royal Marines. This might have scuppered his chance, though I have not discovered the outcome. I also learnt after our return that two Scandinavian climbers who had passed through our camp one morning and had talked to everyone had both died the next day near the summit of the nearby mountain.

The third, now British Exploring Society, expedition was a Dangoor Next Generation very special one to Iceland. It was only three weeks in length, and was for young people of both sexes with either mental or physical disabilities. Apart from blisters, and despite my worries, there were no medical or psychiatric problems at all. The selection after the preceding trial camp in the Lake District had obviously been successful. I have since discovered that in nearly a century of the society organising expeditions that at 79 years old I was their oldest leader.

The other young person expedition that I have done as the medical officer, and as ornithologist, was with the Brathay Foundation to the Faeroe Islands in 1980. To be selected for an overseas expedition, the young boys and girls had to have successfully completed a shorter expedition in Britain. This has the advantage that all the candidates applying for the overseas expeditions had to a marked degree already proven their ability and fitness. We all had various small lacerations from the birds that we were ringing but no more serious problems. The only near-medical problem was me! On the way out we decided to move from our forward camp back to the base camp carrying all our personal gear and the equipment in one march. This was 20km (13 miles) in length, with climbs and descents of more than 1,200m (about 4,000ft). We started with packs of between 60lb and 70lb each, but as several of the twelve-person team were struggling, parts of their packs were loaded onto mine. When I arrived, very exhausted, my pack was weighed at 112lbs (50.8kg). I did take a couple of days to recover.

The Antarctic and the Falkland Islands

On a visit in 2003 we experienced three days of winds of storm force 10 and above. There were several injuries on the boat, including a serious hand injury to one of the passengers. The Croatian doctor on board asked for my advice on the injuries on several occasions. When the boat reached the Falklands Islands I took the Irishman with the crushed finger to the hospital. I was then asked to assist at the operation to repair the damage. This was several days later, and the repair was less than ideal. It was unfortunate that I did not do the operation.

* * *

I have also been on expeditions to Senegal, The Gambia, Kenya and Australia. The only person with a real medical problem was Vivian in the far north-west of Australia when she was bitten by a centipede that had got into her sleeping bag. This was extremely painful, and also worrying as we did not initially know the cause of the bite and feared it could have been a snake, until it – with much reduced poison – bit me. It was then caught, identified and despatched.

Occasional Advice and Help

In 1997 we had been touring southern Africa with very long-term South African friends, John and Margaret Kinvig. As we crossed into Zimbabwe, we saw recent skid marks on the road and came across a car in a ditch. There were unfortunately two dead bodies in the car. When the police arrived, all that was possible was for me to confirm their deaths.

I have been involved in giving first aid or advice in nine countries and in three aeroplanes. This advice often occurred when transport or sporting accidents occurred near me. None was life-threatening and my help was in the initial phase and ensuring that either recovery had occurred or the emergency services had attended. The three occasions on which I had been asked for help on an aeroplane were more worrying. No skilled assistance would have been available, and often the emergency equipment that is carried is insufficient. The first case was when Vivian and I were flying from London to Dubai. An elderly lady from the Far East, who was travelling on her own, had what was an obvious heart attack, but remained conscious. There was no alternative to removing her from the plane in Dubai, but we did feel sorry for her, being in a country on her own and with no language in common. On the continuation of that flight a young lad had a severe tummy ache. This time a doctor was not called over the speakers. The hostess simply arrived and asked me to see him. It was not an appendicitis, and after administering a painkiller, the plane carried on. The third occasion was on a plane flying back from Sri Lanka, when a lady had lost consciousness. This time a young English doctor who had worked for Médecins sans Frontières also responded. The patient's husband explained that his wife had had awful diarrhoea and vomiting, and she was severely dehydrated. An intravenous drip was inserted, and she regained consciousness but needed to be kept horizontal. After considerable discussion, the captain agreed that we would put her behind some seats, which would give her protection in the event of a crash on landing. All went well and at the captain's request, all passengers remained in their seats after landing at Heathrow until the patient had been removed by paramedics. To my surprise not a single passenger stood up. The other doctor and I received a letter of thanks signed by the captain – but no offer of a free flight or an upgrade in the future! I have heard of American doctors giving first aid or advice, and then sending in a bill.

There is the story of the request on a flight for an anaesthetist to make themselves known. When one volunteered, they were asked to go into the first-class section. Asking about the problem, they were told that there was an orthopaedic surgeon there who needed his reading light adjusting. This joke is appreciated by all doctors and nurses except orthopaedic surgeons and anaesthetists, as it was a little too close to the truth in many operating theatres.

Summary

My overseas work was made possible as the NHS gave me two weeks a year for study leave, and this could include teaching or going to conferences. I was also allowed two weeks' special leave in Britain, but which included examining overseas. I also had six weeks of holiday a year, and for many years would have two weeks' skiing with the family, and the other four weeks working or teaching overseas.

Including disasters and wars and other work mentioned elsewhere, I have operated in twenty-five countries, taught/lectured on medical subjects in twenty-nine countries and been on expeditions in fifteen countries. It has been an interesting selection. However, despite these travels I have only been officially licensed as a doctor in Britain, Australia (the state of Victoria only) and, incredibly, South Sudan. No one else was apparently bothered!

Chapter 10

Teaching, Examining, Media and Medico-Legal Work

Teaching

I have been teaching since the age of 9. It started with boys and girls in my form at primary school, helping them to read and write, and also at cubs when I became a sixer. As a teenager I was teaching scouts, and at Leeds and Cambridge Universities, and for the Youth Hostels Association, I taught sailing.

My serious teaching started in my second year of research at Cambridge, where I was demonstrating physics in the Cavendish Laboratory, supervising chemistry at St Catharine's College, and teaching maths at the Cambridge Technical College. What one will do to earn money! – but it was enjoyable. Two years as an assistant lecturer, followed by one year after promotion to lecturer in chemical engineering, then followed at the University of Surrey. And this continued on a part-time basis during my first year back at Cambridge to read medicine. I followed this as a full-time demonstrator in anatomy at the University of Zambia. The remainder of this section is a summary of my part-time teaching in medical subjects.

My first spell of tutoring anatomy at Oxford was to the undergraduate medical students of St Edmund Hall in my third year of clinical studies. I cannot remember how this post came about, but I do not remember applying for it. Then on to my house surgical post in Cambridge. I was recruited by Dr Gordon Wright, the senior director of studies in medicine at Clare College. I became the supervisor in anatomy for Newnham College and Trinity Hall for that academic year. Back to Oxford the next year as an SHO, and an immediate request to be a part-time demonstrator in the anatomy laboratory. I think there must have been a hot telephone wire between the two universities! I was also asked to teach neuroanatomy. I was very pleased to add this to my subjects, as I was at the time still considering neurosurgery as a career. This had an interesting sequel.

Trainee psychiatrists, all qualified for several years, were required to take the examination of the Diploma in Psychiatric Medicine, and neuroanatomy was a compulsory part of this. Of all the teaching that I have done in my life, teaching psychiatrists was the hardest of all. It was a very welcome relief when the undergraduates returned a month later. In this same period I also taught anatomy to student radiographers – much easier than psychiatrists as they were actively interested. Somebody must have discovered that I had taught physics at Cambridge, and I was asked to teach trainee radiologists about radioactivity. I had moved to the accident surgery post when a similar experience to my recruitment as a track doctor occurred (*see* Chapter 7). I had been seeing patients at the front desk in turn, and despite calling next several times, one very distinguished gentleman just sat there. When all the other waiting patients had been seen, he came over asked if I would mind if he asked me a question. I was becoming rather worried, but his question very simply was would I please tutor the medical students at Christ Church? With pleasure, I said – considerably relieved. And even before term had started I was also asked to tutor Magdalen College students. I used the undergraduate rooms in two of the most beautiful colleges in Oxford, and they were interesting groups to teach. The system in Oxford was totally different from Cambridge. On returning from the long vacation they sat the first, and an important, exam of the year – and hopefully they had been working over their holiday. I thought it a very unfriendly system. At least in Cambridge there may have been work during a long vacation if one had one – but then there was a clear holiday for travelling. I remember three of my students in particular. One extremely pleasant Magdalen man sadly became involved in drugs and was thrown out of the College. The second one had been a junior international rugby player, but exams were not his thing. Having been told to read the question papers carefully, he answered four instead of five questions. He was the only one of the 200+ students to whom I taught anatomy who failed. He did retake the exam and is now a GP. The third one that I remember was extremely clever, and after our first tutorial said that anatomy was very simple and very boring. Three weeks later he came up to me and said that he was now finding it a challenge and was interested. I am still not sure whether my brilliant teaching had challenged him, or my teaching was so bad that he had not understood it and needed to do some extra work!

When I was working at the Birmingham Accident Hospital, and particularly with a trauma team, there was a steady flow of medical students.

Teaching, Examining, Media and Medico-Legal Work

I found it surprising that although in a world-famous hospital, few were interested, and also how appalling was their lack of anatomical knowledge. This appeared to be endemic amongst Birmingham students and graduates at the time as I had successive housemen who did a venous cut-down – a very basic operation – on the wrong side of the ankle. I suggested that they should have looked at their own ankles to work out the anatomy which is externally visible and very obvious. At Nottingham and Newcastle I taught students who were a relief after Birmingham. The last medical students that I taught were when I was a consultant. At Stoke Mandeville we had small groups of students from King's College, London, and from the University of Grenada, who were attached to us for two to three weeks. There were also two elective students from South Africa. These were Tanya and Suzanne Kinvig, who were the daughters of old friends and who stayed with us for three months, and spent time in the hospital and in general practice. They marked the end of my teaching of medical students. From then on most of my medical teaching has been of doctors or of first aiders from St John and the Scouts.

At Stoke Mandeville one of the extra posts that I took on was as the Royal College of Surgeons tutor. This was partly an advisory post to young surgeons in training, but I also planned and ran mock membership examinations with my consultant colleagues. The other teaching that we did on almost a yearly basis was a study half-day for ambulance, police and fire personnel. These grew in popularity and were also attended by accident department staff from our hospital and from other local hospitals.

In Chapter 7 I mentioned the requirement to pass the Advanced Trauma Life Saving (ATLS) course and being asked to become an instructor. Having passed the instructor course, I have now taught on more than 120 courses in Cambridge, Oxford, Imperial College, Chelsea and Westminster, Birmingham, the Isle of Wight, Peterborough, Poole and North Wales.

Where working is concerned, many years ago I was advised

If you can – do.
If you can't do – teach.
And if you can't teach – teach teachers.

I am luckily still wanted both for teaching and for teaching teachers. I think that I have to accept that my time 'doing' as a surgeon is now past, except in emergencies. Teaching keeps me up to date, enables me to put something back into the system, to talk to young doctors and to my colleagues, and is socially very pleasant.

Examining

I have discovered over the years that examining is very different from teaching. The first examining that I did was in the Scouts for the various tests and badges. I remember one of my Scout colleagues, Bob Provis, was extremely upset when I failed him, I now realise quite unjustifiably, as he could not tell me the Latin name of a star constellation. I can still remember that his failure was due to not knowing that the Great Bear was called *Ursa Major*.

It is interesting that one is taught to teach, but almost never is one taught to examine. The next examining that I did was marking 'A' level chemistry papers. There was an examiners' meeting at Leicester University before we started, but marking the papers was purely a matter of having the correct words in the answers. Some of the papers I was marking were from Singapore, and I remember one candidate who produced not only all the correct answers, but also gave alternative methods of solving the problems. However, because not all of the words required were present, although his overall paper was worthy of a good degree in first-year chemistry, he only scored a 'B'. The marking had to be done in a short space of three weeks, and was extremely boring. It did, however, pay well, and paid for my skiing trip of that year. I did not repeat the experience.

I did no further examining until I was a lecturer in engineering. The difference here was that I also had to set the examination questions in my subject. These were unfortunately not checked, and one year I set a question that could not be properly answered without the candidates making an assumption about a missing piece of information. Remarkably no one noticed.

All written examinations up to this time were before the days of multiple choice questionnaires (MCQs). There is no doubt that MCQs make examining much easier, with two major advantages. Firstly there is no problem interpreting the candidate's writing, and secondly it is much more rapid to mark. It does, though, have two distinct disadvantages. The first, as I have discovered, is that the questions are much more difficult to set, and secondly if there is any doubt when the answer has two close possibilities, it is not possible for this to be made obvious by discussion.

Teaching, Examining, Media and Medico-Legal Work

Up to this time, with the exception of my Scouting experience, all of my examining had been done by written papers. In medicine now, as well as the written papers or MCQs, viva voce examinations are nearly always part of any test. I can see a very good reason for this, particularly for a surgeon. An attempt to assess a candidate's response to being under pressure is part of a viva examination. In many careers there is time to think about one's answers to problems, but in surgery this time may not be available in the middle of an operation. Working safely and competently under pressure, rather than with perfect knowledge, may be of more importance, and certainly a viva examination can indeed be regarded as working under pressure.

I had been a consultant for several years when I noticed a request in the *Bulletin* of the Royal College of Surgeons of England for people to apply to be an examiner for the Fellowship examination. It said that general surgeons and orthopaedic surgeons were preferred. I decided that plastic surgery would also be relevant on the board of examiners. I heard nothing. Some months later in 1994 I was at a conference in Glasgow, and at the dinner I found myself sitting next to Mr Bill Reid. He was the plastic surgery consultant who was the Director of the Burns unit in Glasgow. Somehow examining came into our conversation, and I told him about my application. Nothing further was said at the time, but about three weeks later a letter came from the College in Glasgow asking me to be an examiner. With great pleasure I accepted.

In the 1980s there were four colleges of surgeons in Britain, in London, Edinburgh, Glasgow and Ireland. In theory, a Fellowship from any of the colleges was equivalent, but I am sure that the college relevant to where one was working was on occasions given priority at interviews. The College in Glasgow was different from the other three in that the Royal College of Surgeons and Physicians of Glasgow was a unified body, but the examinations were different, and either the RCS or the RCP letters after one's name were determined by the relevant examination. For my services in 2004 I was awarded the Fellowship of the Royal College of Surgeons of Glasgow to add to my English Fellowship.

In the 1990s there was some confusion in that there were two levels of the Fellowship examination and qualification. At any time four years or longer after one's qualification one could take the Fellowship in surgery. This examination could incorporate any of the branches of surgery. In 1985 at the end of one's specialist training one could then take a new second Fellowship in one's own specialty. One then acquired the letters

FRCS general or FRCS plastic etc. after one's name. This continued for some years and was then changed so that the first examination could be taken three years or more after qualification, and the letters MRCS were then attached after one's name. The next change was in 2004, when the examiners from all four of the Royal Colleges were amalgamated, and one could then examine for any of the colleges. I continued examining until 2010, and examined in ten centres in Scotland, England and the United Arab Emirates.

On my appointment as an examiner for the Royal College of Surgeons of Glasgow I had to attend two examinations as an observer before I was allowed to examine. However, there was no formal teaching of examining technique at that stage. I remember watching an examiner trying to drag some rather abstruse information from a candidate. The candidate clearly did not know the information, but the examiner would not stop and alter his question. I thought that he was very unfairly failed. During the sixteen years that I was an examiner for the Royal Colleges of Surgeons the examinations did change and to some extent improve. The most sensible change was that three topics had to be included in any viva. The next change was to give a list of twelve topics from which the examiner selected three. The great advantage of that system was that one could ask a mid-line question to start with, and if the candidate did well, then a more difficult question could follow. If the candidate did poorly, then a more simple question would be asked. At each part of the examination two examiners were present, and after a discussion a pass/fail decision was made. The next change was that specific questions only were asked, and this took away the examiner's ability to try to assess candidates who were either above or below the mid-line. This was extremely boring for the examiner, and it was at this point that I gave up examining for the Fellowship as I thought that it could equally well have been done by a robot. These changes were all instituted on the requirements of education 'experts' with the purpose of making the examination 'more fair'. I personally think that we should have ignored much of this advice as it became almost impossible to put the candidate under pressure, and this to me was a very negative change.

A very different form of examining that I have done only once was when I was asked to be the external examiner for an Oxford DPhil thesis. Having to read a complete thesis and then to criticise it was very different. The thesis was about damage caused to skin and the biological reaction to the damage. It was therefore only partly in my field, and my only criticisms were mathematical – which were much more in my field. The internal examiner and I passed the candidate with some minor corrections.

Another form of examining that I did, and continue to do, was to review scientific papers submitted to journals for publication, and also textbooks before publication. I have done this for seven journals including the *British Medical Journal* and the *Lancet*. One of the papers that I reviewed for *Tropical Doctor* was a very useful piece of research, and my job for that one was to turn it into good English.

The final surgical examining that I have been involved with for the past thirteen years is for the Advanced Trauma Life Support (ATLS) course. This was a three-day course for doctors only, and consisted of one day of lectures and two days of discussions, and then the candidates examined mock patients, during which time they could be questioned at any point. This was followed by a multiple-choice paper. In the most recent edition three years ago, the day of lectures was moved on-line. I personally found this made the course less interesting. As well as being of advantage to recently qualified doctors looking for promotion through the ranks, the qualification is a requirement for consultants in the relevant specialties of Accident and Emergency, plastic surgery, and orthopaedic surgery. Success is at two levels, firstly a simple pass or fail, but those who pass sufficiently well can be recommended to become future instructors provided they have had sufficient experience since qualifying as a doctor. These instructor candidates then attend a two-day course which includes both input from educational experts, and also watching, and then commenting on, the examination of the mock patient. Since qualifying as an instructor, I have taught on six of these instructor candidate courses. When examining the mock patient, the instructors act as the candidates. We are asked to attempt to be borderline, and I think we all find it difficult not to do the examination properly. It is suggested that we either miss something important, or even make a deliberate mistake. The ideal instructor is apparently successful when one instructor candidate passes them and one fails them. I managed this only once. The important thing about the ATLS course is that no one can become an instructor until they have also passed the course on how to instruct and how to examine. This is a surprisingly rare requirement in most examinations.

Since becoming a consultant, the vast majority of my teaching has been of doctors and not of medical students. At no stage in my career have I had to examine medical students for their final examinations. I can see that it would be quite difficult to assess the level of a pass needed to be a safe doctor, without perfection being required.

Other examining that I have done is in first aid for St John Ambulance, and away from medicine completely, examining sailors for their ability both to sail and to be safe at sea, and also of biologists training as bird-ringers. Over the years of examining that I have done, the oral part has been particularly interesting and worthwhile. Marking papers is very much less rewarding. As long as I am wanted, I will continue to examine for sailing and for ornithology.

Media

As a medical student or as a doctor one is not taught or given advice about how to deal with the media. As I said in Chapter 6, the Bradford Stadium Fire disaster very rapidly gave me practice. My next meeting with the media was in South Africa, and again the discussion was about Bradford and disasters. In South Africa in 1987 there was a radio programme which was very similar to 'Today' on the BBC. It comprised a series of short interviews about current news, and once a week there was a 15-minute interview instead of the usual 1 to 2 minutes. I presume that the South African radio station discovered about my visit from the pharmaceutical company which had arranged and funded it. I do know that the person who interviewed me was absolutely brilliant. We had had a 1-minute conversation before the interview started, and it then went on for 15 or 20 minutes with him asking sensible questions, and not interfering with my answers. How that differs from so many of the 'Today' interviewers. By chance about four days later we were travelling in a car with the radio on, and my interview was being broadcast. It turned out that they had selected it for the 15-minute slot.

On the burn unit at Stoke Mandeville in 1988 there was an elderly lady with severe arthritis. She had been in a bath filling with hot water. Unfortunately the water was extremely hot and was scalding her, but because of her arthritis she could not easily reach the tap to turn it off. She was quite seriously burned over some 25 per cent of her body. I received a phone call from Gavin Campbell from the 'That's Life' BBC programme. In general, 'That's Life' was a light-hearted review, but once or twice a year they included more serious items about accidents, their prevention and treatment. On this particular programme they wished to discuss the problem that in most houses the hot water temperature was not controlled, but should have been. I do not know how they knew about my specific patient,

Teaching, Examining, Media and Medico-Legal Work

but she agreed to be interviewed by Gavin, who came down with a photographer to Stoke Mandeville to talk to her, and to me.

The show was to be televised a few weeks later, and Vivian and I were invited to the recording. This was in the Shepherd's Bush Green theatre (later to become the Shepherd's Bush Empire). Interestingly, the recording of the show started an hour before it was due to be televised. I assume that this was so that any errors, bad language or disasters could be edited out, but still gave the idea of spontaneity. All went well with the presentation of the excess temperature of the hot water, in which I had a small input on screen. At the end of the show Vivian and I were invited to join the cast and the producer for a meal in a local restaurant, where I met for the first time Esther Rantzen and her husband Desmond Wilcox. It was a very short meeting with Esther, and a long and interesting discussion with Desmond, with whom I was very impressed. Gavin Campbell's wife Liz was also there, and that was the first of several meetings with her. Also present were two or three of the other main presenters of the show.

When this programme was finished, Gavin asked me to look out for any patient who had been burned in an accident which could have an important message for everybody. Over the next few months we admitted several patients who had been burned because of a barbecue incident. This was normally caused by pouring an inflammable liquid onto a barbecue that was thought to be out. After a discussion with one of these patients, and with their agreement, I phoned Gavin. He was instantly interested and came back to Stoke Mandeville with his photographer to interview both the patient and me. When the show was broadcast it included a fireman in full protective gear throwing half a cup of petrol onto a barbecue. It was very impressive, particularly when shown in slow motion. Very unfortunately, even with his protective gear, the fireman suffered minor burns. The lesson was very obvious. Again my wife and I joined the team for the subsequent dinner.

Following these shows, it was clear that Gavin Campbell was interested in injuries causing burns, and as I was setting up the research trust at this stage, I asked him if he would become a trustee. He very kindly agreed to do this and his input through his media connections was extremely useful. There was a discussion about both of us doing a London marathon to raise funds. I am not sure if I'm grateful or not, but he was injured and decided that he would not be able to do a marathon that year.

My next two interviews were on the radio about local incidents, and the third one was on the BBC World Service talking about the initial treatment of a burn when it occurred. My first overseas broadcast was in Greece in 1992 when I was there for their petroleum refinery disaster (*see* Chapter 6). This was of course in English, and whether a translation was given I do not know. In 1993 when I was in India co-organising the first Indian national microsurgery course, I gave an introduction to microsurgery and why it was needed, on Indian national television.

My next connection with the media came about through somebody whom I had briefly met doing 'That's Life'. She asked me if I would be the medical adviser to a series of programmes called 'The Paranormal World of Paul McKenna'. I was involved in two of the programmes, in which a very unusual Ukrainian man demonstrated abnormal physical attributes. He could stay underwater for 15 minutes without breathing, and this was almost reproduced on the programme but it turned out that the water was colder than expected, and this made him shiver. This used up extra energy and oxygen, and he failed in his record bid by two minutes. He was also able to ignore severe electric shocks. My contribution was to comment on the science, and not to have to resuscitate him, for which I was very grateful.

There followed a series of interviews on national and local television and radio about topical subjects such as firework injuries, fire-safe cigarettes and garage fires, as well as the role of plastic surgery and new treatments. The series 'Siege Doctors' about our work in Sarajevo has been described in Chapter 6.

My next major contribution was when I was invited to the Philippines by the British Ambassador Alan Collins, who was heading a campaign to try to reduce the very common burn injuries from fireworks. I did three programmes on their national television.

Stoke Mandeville Hospital was very unusual, and in the United Kingdom, unique. It incorporated the world famous spinal injuries unit and a nationally famous burns and plastic surgery unit, both within a small district general hospital. This caused some resentment; for instance the NHS awards for excellence were preferentially given to the two specialist unit doctors, and secondly we were approached more by the media for opinions and information. I remember at one point a senior consultant colleague asked me why I was always on television. My response was that I did not ask to be on television, but that I was asked to be on television. Over thirty-four years I have been involved in seventeen television appearances and twenty-four radio interviews in seven countries.

Teaching, Examining, Media and Medico-Legal Work

I think a lot would be gained by having the facility for all doctors to be briefed on dealing with the media. I am not sure whether this would be better done for medical students, junior doctors, or on becoming a consultant. With the increase in local radio and television stations, there must be an increasing chance for a doctor being asked for an interview. The first time that it happened to me, with no previous experience, although after many years of teaching, it was still a surprise. Looking back, I was extraordinarily lucky that it was Kate Adie, and even luckier that it was a face-to-face interview and not talking into a camera. In my experience talking to a camera when one is in a room with only a camera operator present is much more difficult than talking to another person. And when it is a radio interview, particularly over a telephone or similar, it is even more difficult as one cannot even see a face to see how the interviewer is reacting.

Of course, the actual technique of speaking can be practised, and there are major advantages in doing so. It sounds very obvious, but one only has to watch television or listen to the radio to realise that the basic rule of speaking slowly and clearly does not always apply, even among politicians. My advice will always be that it is wise to answer the question, and then shut up. Very often the interviewee just wishes to keep talking, and this automatically invites interruption. This appears to be particularly true of politicians! One then has the situation where no question is actually answered before an interruption by the person doing the interview. I personally find this extremely objectionable. It is also much more satisfactory if the interview is being broadcast live as it then cannot be edited. An interview that is not live and has been edited by the interviewer or their producer may give a completely different impression from what one had wished to say. Listening to the radio or watching television, one slowly realises that there is normally a goody and a baddy on any subject. The advantage that a doctor normally has is that he or she is the goody. Being the goody, as I have been throughout my media career, has made my life with the media very much easier.

Another piece of advice I would strongly give is not to be interviewed about a subject unless one really knows what one is talking about. On one occasion I was phoned by the BBC and asked to do an interview on the cosmetic surgery of the famous American pop-star Michael Jackson. Having no interest whatsoever in Michael Jackson, and very little knowledge or experience of any relevant cosmetic surgery, my answer to the request was, 'Who is Michael Jackson?' At the other end of the telephone there was a silence, and a slow intake of breath. 'I think I am talking to the wrong person,' said the potential interviewer. I said, 'I totally agree with you. Goodbye.'

Medico-Legal Work

There can be few doctors who do not encounter the legal profession at some time in their professional lives. This may be in the coroner's court, giving evidence at a trial or when there have been problems either with work, with patients or with colleagues.

The legal profession in England is different from most parts of the world with the exception of some Commonwealth countries which have in general used the English legal system. Qualified lawyers are divided into solicitors and barristers. On both sides of the profession there is specialisation into criminal, civil or family law. There is also the separate branch of coroners, who are normally solicitors working as a coroner part-time, but they may also be full-time. In their professional life doctors were able to work as coroners until 2013, but this is no longer an option. Doctors may also work as police surgeons, which again may be full- or part-time, as medical legal experts, or in tribunals.

On a personal level, my introduction to a court was being fined after I had been caught speeding by radar at night in London. Some years later I was summonsed for a parking offence in Oxford, for which I personally went to court as I thought the signs totally misleading. Needless to say, I was told the signs were perfectly legal and I was fined. I was then extremely upset when all of the signs were changed within months. Unfortunately I could not afford the cost of an appeal. I had two other summonses for being caught speeding, one of which was in Zambia with probably the only radar set in the whole country.

Within the medical profession legal work can be either civil or criminal. Anyone suing their employer, a company, a doctor or the National Health Service is normally a civil case. Murder, grievous bodily harm or any other similar illegal occurrences are criminal cases. The doctors most involved in civil litigation are Accident and Emergency consultants, orthopaedic consultants and plastic surgery consultants. Plastic surgery patients will normally have an obvious injury or a scar. The very much more difficult cases which are seen by orthopaedic surgeons are those with, for instance, a whiplash injury to their neck. There are no physical or x-ray findings to define the severity of such an injury, but it is remarkable how some patients become much better as soon as the case in court is finished.

Teaching, Examining, Media and Medico-Legal Work

When I became a consultant as a plastic surgeon I rapidly became involved in writing medical reports on patients who were suing other people, employers or companies. In the 1980s there was no formal training qualification required before examining patients or their records, and then writing a medico-legal report. The request would come from the patient's solicitor, and for the civil work the doctor involved was normally the one who had examined or treated the patient.

I wrote many hundreds of reports during my consultant career, often as many as two a week. For every hundred civil reports that I wrote, ninety-nine would be settled out of court with no further input from me. The remaining 1 per cent that went to court required me to take a day off work from my leave time. I would then attend court, normally in London, only to find that 50 per cent of those cases were then settled out of court when everybody was there and ready to go into court. This meant that I had lost a day of my holiday time, but I was at least paid for it. The first few times I was in court were extremely stressful as I had had no formal training in the subject. It became clear that many of the patients deserved compensation for the accidents in which they had been involved. There were, however, many for whom compensation was inappropriate and who had been advised to sue by personal injury lawyers. Many of these lawyers recruited their customers by advertising or by telephoning people at random. There has also been an increasing number of people who have sued hospitals since medical insurance cover was taken over by the NHS in the 1980s. These cases are often for very minor problems that may or may not have occurred. Prior to this, all doctors had medical insurance cover through companies such as the Medical Defence Union or the Medical Protection Society. The MDU has always taken the line that unless malpractice was evident, the company would defend the accused doctor in court. Solicitors knew this and would only take on obvious malpractice cases. Since the change, it has been an absolute disaster for the NHS. Because of the cost of defending any action, the health service basically pays out if the sum claimed is less than a few hundred pounds, whether there was any fault or not, and some injury lawyer solicitors know this only too well.

I well remember one case. A patient of mine and her husband were building their own house. On a very cold day the pre-mixed concrete arrived for the foundations, and some of it went into her boots. This caused a chemical burn which I treated at Stoke Mandeville. It healed a few weeks later but left her with some scarring. She was suing the company for not warning her that concrete is dangerous. After his introductory questions, the junior barrister defending the company asked me, 'Tell me doctor, how does concrete burn?' I told him the chemistry of the reaction. I could almost see the next question that was coming, which was, 'You are, of course, an expert in chemistry, Doctor?' To which my reply was, 'I have been a university lecturer in chemical engineering.' I could see the judge trying to smother a laugh. The case finished and my patient received some damages.

I avoided all but one case asking me to be a witness against my colleagues when a patient had been unhappy with the result of their surgery. The vast majority of these were cosmetic (aesthetic) surgery which was very definitely not my area of expertise. The one case that I did handle was a burn case.

Criminal work is very different. Any doctor may be required to attend as a witness of fact, or they may be present as an expert witness. As a doctor my only appearance in a criminal court as a witness of fact was in Bridgwater, Somerset and concerned a patient whom I had seen when I was working as a casualty officer in Taunton Hospital. He had had a scalp laceration and bruising. The Crown Prosecution Service barrister asked me whether this could have been caused by being hit on his head with a stick. My answer was yes. The defending counsel then asked me whether it could have been caused by him falling over and hitting his head on a pavement edge. Again my answer had to be yes. Looking back afterwards with years of experience, the injuries could have been differentiated, and in fact it turned out from a witness that he had been hit on the head with a stick.

In criminal cases the decision as to whether to sue a person or company is the responsibility of the Director of Public Prosecutions. In the 1980s the DPP might employ an expert, and the defence could employ a second expert. Both examined the records and the patient and wrote reports. Following the reports, if the DPP took the case to court, then it would be normal for the medical experts to attend court to be questioned by the various counsels. In theory the experts are neutral and should not be supporting the side that hired them. This is actually quite difficult, and the system has now changed in that only one expert witness is hired and thus can more easily be seen to be neutral.

My experience started with one of my patients, a young boy, who had been intentionally burned by his mother's partner. To any normal person this is horrific, but it is more common than expected. A scientific paper from Manchester in the 1970s said that in 14 per cent of the children who were admitted with burns, intention was proven or very likely to have happened. In my first case my evidence was accepted, and the man went to prison for grievous bodily harm (GBH). Other cases followed and I began to get the reputation for success in getting offenders committed to prison. The DPP started to ask me to be their expert regularly around England.

On one occasion two South African lawyers visited my unit and asked me to fly to South Africa for a case. The problem was that as I was being hired by them, they expected me to totally back their client. I told them that that was not how the system worked in England. Clearly somebody else whom they had approached had told them the same thing, and they departed without an expert witness who would do as he or she was told.

Three particular cases I remember well. In the first, from an examination of the burn distribution, a young child had very obviously been intentionally burned. The problem was that the story given by each of the parents did not explain the pattern of the burning. It was therefore decided by the DPP that it was not possible to accuse one of them, and the offender escaped justice. It still upsets me to this day.

The second case was much more obvious and the mother's boyfriend was clearly guilty. There was a young barrister attempting to defend him. After all the standard questions the case was clearly going against him, and looking very worried he asked, 'Are you 100 per cent sure that this could not have happened any other way?' Before I could answer the Judge said, 'Nothing is 100 per cent certain in medicine, is it, doctor?' 'Only death, my Lord,' was my answer.

The third case was an extremely unfortunate one for several reasons. A 14-year-old girl of Nigerian origin had very severe hot water burns from which she died. It had been suggested by the hospital that the burns could have been intentional. I was asked to visit the house in London where it had happened with the solicitor involved in the defence of her mother. We were shown the bath, and noted that there was no plug present. Her father told us that in Nigeria no one had a full bath, but used it for showering only. He had no explanation as to what could have happened, but had noticed that when she was found the bath was full of very hot water, which was overflowing as the drain was blocked. I noticed in the pathologist's report that severe bruising on the back of the scalp had been noticed. A possible explanation was that she had slipped in the bath and knocked herself out as she fell. The outlet could have been plugged by a flannel or something else, and she had been burned by the rising hot water. She was taken to the local hospital, but died during transfer to the regional burn unit. In court the pathologist accepted that the story and the findings were possible, and admitted that she was puzzled by the bruising. The mother was discharged, but as she left the court she was rearrested as an illegal immigrant.

In my last year as an expert witness I was involved in two murder cases, two attempted murder cases and three GBH cases.

It is relatively common for a doctor, and especially a pathologist, to appear in the coroner's court. The role of coroner in England goes as far back as 1194, and is mentioned in the Magna Carta of 1215. The role was originally as a tax gatherer, but developed into an independent judicial officer whose duty was to establish the cause of death in cases of sudden, violent or unnatural death. Most deaths do not automatically go to a coroner. If the person is under medical care and their doctor is willing to sign a death certificate, then a coroner can intervene, but rarely does so. This can obviously go wrong, as it did in the case of Dr Harold Shipman, and the system is dependent on the honesty of the doctor concerned. How a death is investigated, and whether it needs to involve a court, is in the judgement of the coroner. They may also, in most cases, decide whether a jury is necessary.

I did appear in one coroner's court as a junior doctor. Four of us had been driving in Lincolnshire and came across a crashed car. Unfortunately there was one dead young lady who had been thrown out of the vehicle. I was summoned to the coroner's court in Lincoln. In my evidence I tried to emphasise that had she been wearing a seatbelt, she would not have been thrown out of the car and would probably have survived. Unfortunately, the coroner failed to pick this up, and apologised to me afterwards for not doing so.

People who die from burns automatically become a coroner's case as the cause is unnatural. In Aylesbury any patient dying in the burn unit at Stoke Mandeville would automatically be referred to the local coroner, Mr Corner. He always asked, in fact legally demanded, that I went to court. He explained to me later that this was so that the relatives could ask me any questions if they wished. In fact, in the sixteen years of my attendances the only responses I had from relatives in the court were their thanks for looking after the person who had died.

When I moved to the Isle of Wight in 2001 I did consider the possibility of becoming an assistant coroner, as I had found the work interesting. I wrote to the coroner, Mr John Matthews, who replied that he was only part-time and did not therefore need an assistant. Having discovered something about my medical and legal background, he did, however, follow it up by asking me in 2007 and subsequently to be an expert witness in appropriate coroner's cases. I was involved with several over the next few years. Two things struck me. Firstly, how superb he was at talking to the relatives when the case had been concluded – a very difficult job. The second thing was how copious were the notes that I had to analyse. Clearly at least half of every package was just a waste of paper, but more importantly was the time spent on the wards filling out irrelevant forms. It struck me as a case of severe management overload. The cases that John sent me were initially in my areas of expertise, but over the years the scope widened. We were obviously speaking the same language. In 2013 John retired, and the new coroner was Mrs Caroline Sumeray. I still had some cases in the pipeline, which I completed, and she did ask me to do a couple more, but then the cases ceased. I wonder if this was because of a disagreement over a diagnosis as to the cause of death. It concerned an elderly lady who was mentally normal and had refused further treatment. She acquired severe pressure sores, which caused her death. Mrs Sumeray considered that this was a case of failure by the doctors and nurses looking after her. I pointed out in court that any adult who is mentally normal has an absolute right to refuse treatment. The coroner eventually agreed with me, but that was the end of new cases and I retired as adviser to the coroner in 2019.

One interesting case that I did handle was an NHS investigation into a hospital in south-east England which had been reported because of unacceptable management of a case. It was about a young (20+) footballer who had been admitted with a fractured leg and left the hospital some weeks later with the leg having been amputated. After reading all the notes and the statements of the doctors involved, I visited the hospital to interview both the doctors and the patient. Amazingly the patient had not thought of suing the hospital, and I suggested that he did so. One junior surgeon was sent for further training.

Summary

Medico-legal work has been both interesting and financially rewarding. It has required a large amount of work, but most of the civil and all the criminal work was, I felt, justified. There have been annoyances, and in particular the volume of irrelevant notes which often appeared, and also the days of my leave that were lost when cases were settled out of court on the doorstep of the Royal Courts of Justice.

My final annoyance has been that the NHS has taken over the medical insurance cover for all hospital work and this has caused the costs to the NHS to rise substantially. It has also caused the experience of trainee surgeons to be limited as management are unwilling to allow them to operate as it may increase the costs further. This is a terribly circular argument as it also means that when a consultant is appointed, their ability is far less than it used to be at that stage – and the costs rise anyway.

My view of some (but by no means all) lawyers can be easily summarised. In Australia there is a plant with sharp prickles facing in the opposite direction from most plant prickles, so that once it gets hold of you it does not let go. It is called the Lawyer Vine (*Smilax australis*) – I wonder why!

Chapter 11

Patients

Remembering former patients has been an interesting experience. Some I remember because they were unusual, some because they were famous, some because of their characters, and some because things went wrong. Of course, I cannot mention the names of patients without their permission, therefore I have given them arbitrary names where appropriate.

* * *

One of the patients that I will never forget was a gentleman from the spinal injuries unit. Mr Smith had been in the services and had had a nasty accident that left him with a fracture of his lumbar spine, and therefore a loss of function and sensation from his mid-abdomen down. This injury had apparently changed his life, not only physically but also mentally, and from being a troublemaker he became a respectable citizen. He had set up a company which involved him driving. One of the problems with spinal injuries is that although the affected limbs are totally paralysed at the beginning, over time the limbs often develop a rigidity which can cause them to suddenly twitch – often quite markedly. This is obviously a major problem when one is driving as it can cause the car to swerve all over the road. Mr Smith therefore came back to the spinal injuries unit and requested that his right leg was amputated above the knee to stop this problem when he was driving. This I did for him without complications and he was extremely pleased with the result.

And then some two years later he returned to the spinal injuries unit because his left leg had developed the same problem, and he requested that this also be removed above the knee. He was admitted for me to do this, but unfortunately on the morning of his operation the anaesthetist was ill and so was my registrar. I therefore went to see Mr Smith to tell him that his operation had to be cancelled. His immediate response was, 'Why? I cannot feel my limbs anyway, so why can you therefore not simply cut it off?' We agreed to go ahead. The operation was already complicated because after his original accident a metal bar had been put into the femur, the thighbone, on that limb. I knew from the x-rays the type of metal pin that had been put in and I had readied the necessary apparatus for removing it. The first amusing part of this story was when he came to the operating theatre, nurses checking him noticed that he had a large arrow drawn on his left leg. This was causing him great amusement, which the nurses could not understand – at which point he pulled back the bedclothes showing them that his other leg was already missing. In considerable embarrassment, they had to point out that it was most important that I operated on the correct leg! I therefore went ahead with the operation. I exposed the end of the pin, but it proved impossible to remove, even with the correct apparatus. The alternative procedure was to saw the metal rod in half. I therefore had sterilised a hacksaw and a quantity of blades. I made the usual incisions in the skin and started sawing. It became clear that this was going to be a difficult job as the rod itself turned out to be titanium and that is a very difficult and tough metal to cut. After using about three of the blades, by which time I was sweating profusely and missing my absent registrar, Mr Smith commented, chuckling gently, 'I can see why surgeons are so well paid! It's quite hard work, isn't it!'

I carried on and eventually all went well and the amputation was completed. Mr Smith was delighted with the result and that was my last contact with him, although I was told that he came back to the spinal unit for normal check-ups afterwards, and always managed to be admitted when there was a royal visitor, and also when Mrs Bush, the wife of the then American President, visited.

* * *

Mr Jones had been a bomber pilot during the war. When his plane had crashed and caught fire, he was the only survivor although very badly burned. He was treated and survived, and after the war led a life in commerce and got married. In 1997 he was celebrating his Golden Wedding anniversary with his wife at a local Indian restaurant. The chef was preparing a special flambé dish for them beside their table and very unfortunately it all fell onto him, causing severe burns to some of the grafted areas on his legs from fifty years earlier. He was a lovely patient and unbelievably phlegmatic: 'Oh well, I've had it all done before.' His new grafts healed without a problem. I never did discover what happened to the chef in the Indian restaurant.

* * *

Patients

Mr Green had been a member of the Royal Air Force Falcons Parachute Display Team and had tragically broken his back. He had been a patient with the Spinal Injuries Unit for several years and had a very successful post-services career. Unfortunately he had badly burnt one foot and lower leg. With no sensation, injuries including burns are common amongst spinally injured patients and need special care as the tissues, and particularly the skin, heal less well than in a patient with normal sensation. I admitted Mr Green, excised the burned areas and put on split skin grafts. All went well and he had 100 per cent healing. Whilst he was with us on the burn unit he told us that when he was parachuting he had painted the words 'Dig Here' on top of his helmet in case of chute failure. Luckily his accident, although very serious, was not as bad as that!

* * *

Mr White was a Special Air Service officer, and after his retirement from the Army was working for an explosives company when a serious explosion caused him to receive severe burns and some bone damage as well. On his admission, we were going to photograph the extent of his injuries, but he objected strongly. We had a long discussion and it became apparent that he did not want a photograph of his face on record. We agreed that we would not show his face, and the photographs were taken. He required three operations over the coming three weeks. He was then discharged and warned about being careful as the skin grafts and the bone repairs were still very fragile. I saw him regularly in the clinic, and after eight weeks he told me that he had just completed a marathon, luckily without damage to his grafts. The SAS are different from normal humans!

* * *

Mr Brown was referred to me as a private patient with very severe recurrent Dupuytren's contractures of his hands. This is a relatively common disease, but can vary enormously in its speed of onset and in its severity. The surgery is often very difficult and special training and experience are required to handle the more difficult cases. The worse of Mr Brown's hands had had two previous operations by a consultant orthopaedic surgeon, but when he returned again the surgeon told him that it was time he was seen by an expert. He told me that his instant reply had been, 'Why didn't you send me to an expert the first time?' It was perhaps not only training in hand surgery that the orthopaedic surgeon needed.

* * *

Horse riders are strongly advised never to wrap the reins around their hands when riding. Unfortunately this advice is not always given when leading a horse. Miss White was 15 when the horse she was leading with the reins wrapped around her hand bucked and completely pulled off her right thumb. When I saw her in casualty it was clear that the thumb remnant was too severely damaged to have any chance of being replanted. I therefore cleaned up and closed the wound. I saw her in the clinic two weeks later. All was well healed and the sutures were removed. The rest of her hand was functioning well, with a full range of movement. I congratulated her on this as she must have exercised it well, despite some discomfort. I then started to tell her about the possibility of markedly improving the future function of her hand by doing a toe to thumb transfer. Miss White was strongly against this but after further explanation her mother was very strongly in favour. They went home to discuss it further, and after a few days my secretary took a phone call with the request to put Miss White on the operating list. There are often difficult decisions to make in surgery. When Miss White was admitted for the transfer, I had to decide whether to tell her about the complications, and even the chance of total failure. I decided that I would discuss this only with her mother. The operation went ahead, and I used Miss White's big toe and some local skin to make her a new thumb in an operation that took about 5 hours. All went well and the new thumb and the remnant of her toe both healed well. She attended physio and occupational therapy and was soon back at school, and within weeks was back in the saddle. Some months later I did a minor correction to the shape of her new thumb, again with success. She came regularly to the clinic, which I would normally do with a trainee surgeon. When they saw her scarred thumb, I would ask them what they thought had been the original injury, and their answers often amused both Miss White and me – and were very rarely correct. She would then slip off her shoe and almost, but not quite, wave her foot with the absent big toe under their noses, when normally the truth would dawn. Miss White became first a secretary and later a nurse.

* * *

Many of my hand surgery patients had rheumatoid arthritis. This is a dreadful and very painful disease, much commoner in women than men. It can affect any joint, but the hands are commonly involved. It causes pain, loss of function and often deformity. They were normally the most lovely patients who had often tolerated the pain for years and were so grateful when the pain was reduced by surgery. They were also some of the patients that we came to know well as the arthritis progressed and further surgery became useful. I remember in particular Mrs Black, a lady of about 60, with severe problems in both wrists. I agreed to an operation and removed the trapezium bone in her worse wrist, which was the main source of her pain, and then reconstructed the wrist. The operation went well. I saw her in the clinic two weeks later to remove the splint and put on a lighter splint, so that she could start exercising the wrist and hand. As soon as the splint was off and she had made the first gentle movements, her immediate reaction was, 'When can you do the other one?' I suggested that we wait a few months whilst she started to use the first one and we could then decide on a date, but this was clearly unacceptable to her and back on the urgent waiting list she went.

* * *

About 40 per cent of my patients, both whilst training and when I was a consultant, had been burned. About 700 people a year then died from burn injuries in the United Kingdom, but many who survived were left with scars and sometimes deformities. Scarring, particularly of the face, can cause psychological problems – sometimes major and sometimes minor. I learned very early on that it was impossible to prejudge the effects of this scarring on people's lives. I remember Mr Scarlet, who ended up with a facial scar about 2 × 3cm in size, and which I would have described as minor. But it was not minor to him, and he gave up his job as a bank manager as he could not face his customers. It was terribly sad. Despite our best research efforts, scars still occur.

* * *

I also remember Mr Blue, a skilled toolmaker who had severe burns to both hands. After several weeks of surgery, physio and occupational therapy, he returned full-time to his job with two fingers missing from one hand and one partly missing from the other. He was a firm favourite of the nurses as they would ask him to come to the unit to talk to appropriate new patients with similar injuries. The psychological problems of scars were often much more difficult than the physical ones.

* * *

In my eighteen months at the Birmingham Accident Hospital I was involved in the care of several hundred burned patients. Several of them still stand out in my memory nearly fifty years later.

One of the patients who had been there for six months when I arrived had been severely injured in the Birmingham bombing in November 1974. He was the first person I met who had been injured in a disaster, and the effects were still with him and would remain so for the rest of his life. That same year two pilots from Middle East Airlines were transferred to us having been burned at Beirut airport in a bomb explosion. I talked to them every day. Unfortunately the elder gentleman died, but the younger survived and returned to Lebanon. I lost contact with him and have often wondered to what type of country he had returned.

Another patient was a 30-year-old lady who had been burned in a house fire. As a junior doctor, one very often has more time to talk to patients, and not only about their medical problems. It turned out that Miss Violet was a prostitute. Unfortunately when we discovered the cause of her persistent high temperature, it turned out to be typhoid fever. That closed the unit to new admissions for about three weeks. It also had an interesting side-effect in that we, the registrars, were sent to all the hospitals that normally sent their burn patients to us, to lecture to the accident departments about burn care. One of the hospitals that I went to was Warwick, and by chance one of the consultants to whom I was lecturing was later one of my examiners for the Fellowship. He even remembered me.

Miss Blue was a 14-year-old lass of West Indian origin and was the most tragic of all my burn patients. She had received relatively minor burns but in her genes she carried those for sickle cell anaemia. She unfortunately had the rare serious type. One of the effects, and especially with other medical problems, is pain, which can be very severe and difficult to treat. Miss Blue suffered terribly. Then her kidneys failed and despite our best efforts she died. It was a sad end for a lovely lass who had been extremely brave throughout.

One patient I can name. Dr (later Professor) Michael Waring and I first met when he was admitted to Stoke Mandeville after a crash on the M1 in 1990. He had been hit from behind, as he always insisted on telling me and everyone else! His car, a glass-fibre Lotus Elan, caught fire and despite his rapid exit, he was badly burned. One of the unexpected things about burned patients is that unless they have a serious inhalation injury, once their pain is controlled they can talk normally and sensibly. In our conversation in the admission ward, Michael asked me where I had trained as a medical student. I told him Cambridge and then Oxford. 'I must have taught you in Cambridge – I hope I taught you well!' was his instant response.

He was with us for about four weeks and needed three operations. As he left, I asked him what he had thought his chance of dying from the burns had been on his admission. 'Dying – what do you mean dying?' His title of doctor was for scientific research and was not medical, and he had had no idea that with his age and the degree of burning he had been on the 30 per cent mortality curve.

We became very good friends, sat on various committees together, and I would regularly visit him in Cambridge. When we were dining at the high table in his college, Jesus College, he would introduce me to everyone as his Sawbones! Unfortunately he died last year of unrelated causes.

Miss Pink was a nurse at one of the private hospitals in which I worked. One day she asked me if she could have a brief talk to me. It turned out that she was extremely upset by the shape of her nose. She was indeed a very attractive young lady, with a rather large nose. I told her what could be done and the potential complications of the operation. She told me that she had saved up her money. The anaesthetist, Richard Bunsell, and I agreed to do her operation at a much reduced rate as she was a nurse, and the hospital also gave her a small reduction. She was therefore admitted, and I reduced the size of her nose. She came back two weeks later for the plaster to be removed. She took one look in the mirror, gave a great smile and in front of the other nurse present in the room wrapped her arms around me to give me a kiss. I was embarrassed and immediately told her to be careful because although the bones in her nose were set, they were not yet completely stable. The nurse who was with me was highly amused. This was an interesting example of cosmetic or aesthetic surgery. Miss Pink had been born with the nose, which had always upset her since being a young teenager. In half an hour of operating I solved the problem for her. The line between necessary and aesthetic surgery is often quite narrow. A minor cleft lip causes almost no functional problems for a child, and similarly a lady who has had a breast removed for cancer can be enormously improved psychologically by a reconstruction. In neither of these cases would one think that the operation should not be on the National Health Service.

Another similar patient was Mr Purple. Dr Ian Wood was the psychiatrist who looked after my burn patients with psychological problems. After some months he asked me if I would do bat ear corrections on one of his inpatients in the psychiatric hospital. He had been an inpatient for some fifteen years. His problem was relatively minor in that he was able to work during the daytime, but he could not live outside the hospital at night because people 'were looking at him'. On examination, he had relatively minor sticking-out ears, and I was unconvinced that an operation would help to any major degree. However, Ian Wood had been very helpful to me and I therefore agreed that I would correct the patient's ears under local anaesthetic. When the bandage came off his head two weeks later, he was delighted and within a few weeks Ian told me that he had stopped being an inpatient in the psychiatric hospital and was living a normal life. An operation which probably cost the NHS a few hundred pounds saved many tens of thousands of pounds. I am delighted that I did this on the NHS, but it was aesthetic surgery, as certainly his ears did not work any better when they were pinned back into a normal position.

* * *

In a long clinical life there are always disasters. I was extremely upset when a 12-year-old lad was admitted with about 15 per cent deep burns. He had had a major heart and lung condition for some years and was on the waiting list for a heart/lung transplant. Because of his problem he severely felt the cold, and to warm himself up had got too close to a fire and accidentally set his clothes alight. I discussed this case with Richard Bunsell, the anaesthetist. We knew that with his other problems, if the burns became infected and he became septic it would be fatal. His only chance of survival was to do early surgery on the burns, excise the dead tissue and apply a skin graft. I discussed this with his mother, and she agreed. Tragically, in the middle of the operation his heart failed and he arrested. Despite our efforts, this was untreatable. I went to the burn unit to tell his mother. She, in fact, finished up trying to console me. She was an extremely brave lady who said that she knew that her son's chance of survival was almost zero, and had been expecting the terrible news.

A patient who caused me considerable embarrassment was Mrs Brown. She was elderly and had a small cancer on her face. Although clearly not well off, she insisted on having this removed in the private hospital. There were no problems at all with her surgery, but with the cancer that I had removed, the normal procedure was to follow her up at three-monthly intervals for a year and then less often. She returned after three months with no problems. I decided not to send her a bill for the follow-up and arranged to see her again three months later. This time she arrived with a large bottle of whisky for me. Somewhat embarrassed, I thanked her.

Patients

It was a little awkward as I do not drink whisky. Looking back, I should have said so at the time because over the next two or three years, every time she came to see me, another bottle of whisky appeared. Some fifteen years later I have now given them all away to my relatives.

I was also feeling generous when a patient came to see me to have some amateur tattoos removed from his hands. He was a roofer and somewhat scruffily dressed. I offered a cheap price for the tattoos to be removed in my minor ops surgery at home, and a date was arranged. He turned up for his surgery, which took me about 2 hours, in a very elegant Jaguar car and I was slightly suspicious that I had made an over-generous offer. When he came back to have the sutures removed, he was delighted with the result, but I was less delighted as he arrived in an elegant Rolls-Royce. In the discussion that followed, the fact that I needed a little roofing doing came into the conversation. He volunteered to do this, and I said that I would, of course, pay him. Some weeks later he sent some of the team from his large company along, the roofing was done, and I waited for a bill. Despite three reminders, the bill never came, and eventually I received a note saying that it had been permanently lost on its way to me. The tattoo removal was much appreciated by the patient, and the roofing by me.

One day we were doing a sit-down ward round on the burn unit discussing the patients between ourselves before seeing them. That week the hospital was playing host to a young lady from a local school who was considering applying for a medical school place and was attached to various consultants to see what medicine involved. In the middle of the round I had an urgent call to attend the casualty department and made my way rapidly there. Mr Red had been admitted after an agricultural accident, which had torn off his left arm just below his shoulder. He was about 50 years old, and worked on the same farm where a colleague of his had also lost an arm some three years earlier, which Mr Bruce Bailey, my senior colleague, had replaced for him. Mr Red knew that this had not been a great success as far as function was concerned, although it did look cosmetically normal. He therefore declined the idea of having his arm replaced, and from my own experience I agreed with him. Whilst this discussion was going on, the lass from the school was sent along to see what I was doing. The very first patient that she ever saw was on two stretchers, the patient on one and his arm on a second! She sat down rapidly, but after her visit wrote me a letter saying that she still wanted to do medicine! I tidied up Mr Red's stump. Seeing him later in a clinic, I discovered that he had taken a job as a green-keeper on the local golf course, which he had found he could do with his one good arm. I also found out that he was playing golf one-handed and had an amazing handicap of nine. Clearly his decision not to have the arm replaced had been the correct one.

Then there is a patient who still causes me to think 'Phew – that was a near miss.' When I was working in the casualty department in Reading the police brought in a man who had clearly been in a fight and had lacerations on his face. He was very obviously drunk, and the only way that I could suture him was with the police holding him still. I wrote in the notes that 'he had been sutured while the police were holding him down'. When he came back five days later for the sutures to be removed, unfortunately the receptionist gave him his notes. I was seeing another patient at the time, but I noticed him reading his notes and remembered what I had written. When the patient I was seeing departed, the man, carrying his notes, came over towards me. Although it is much commoner now, even in the 1970s doctors in the hospital were occasionally attacked. I thought that this might be about to happen to me, but his reaction was completely unexpected. He apologised profusely for the trouble that he had caused, and explained that he had just had a row with his girlfriend. Would I please forgive him? Definitely.

In my second year as an undergraduate in Cambridge, I trained as a Samaritans counsellor. The majority of the councillors were elderly ladies, and several of them were somewhat eccentric. The people who came to see us or phoned us were called clients and not patients, and some of them were somewhat eccentric. One of these clients was a young lady who was a self-harmer and had multiple scars on her forearms. We met on several occasions and I eventually persuaded her to see a psychiatrist. I arranged an appointment for her with a doctor who was half GP and half psychiatrist. When the young lady came back to me the following week, her very first comment was, 'That woman you sent me to see was more mad than I am.' I could only agree.

Another self-harmer came into the accident service in Oxford when I was an SHO there. She had also been superficially cutting the skin on her forearm. In her case it was still bleeding and to reduce the risk of infection I suggested to the nurses that they should apply iodine. In the 1970s iodine was dissolved in alcohol and it unfortunately stung painfully when applied to cuts. I heard later that she had thought of doing more self-harm on another day and had first phoned casualty to see if I was on duty. Having heard that I was, she delayed her action until the next day. I passed onto my colleagues what I had done, and iodine was again applied.

It cured her of her self-harming. I still debate whether, although effective, this was ethical.

It is sometimes the strange stories that one remembers, rather than the patient. When I was a house officer in Cambridge I saw a man who had cut his right hand with a circular saw. The wound was not too severe and sewing it up was all that was needed. I then asked him how he had done it. He told me he was making coarse sawdust for a local jam manufacturer, which shall remain nameless. The lumpy sawdust would be used to imitate the pips in strawberry jam! I thought he must be pulling my leg – but he assured me that he was not. The things that one learns from patients!

Another story about a cut hand was both more serious and more unfortunate. This patient had started work as an apprentice furniture manufacturer at the age of 15 in one of the famous furniture factories in High Wycombe. Fifty years later, the day that he came to the hospital was his last working day. He told me that he had not been celebrating inappropriately with his workmates but his concentration had wandered and sadly he amputated part of his left index finger. It was too badly damaged to be replaced and all that I could do was close up the wound. That was his first and only injury during the whole of his career.

Chapter 12

Honours and Awards

The honours system in the United Kingdom has over the years been the subject of much debate and frequent upsets. About twenty years ago it became apparent that it was very political, and a position held within a political party, within industry or the military, or a major donation given to a political party, was sufficient to expect an award. Certainly the Order of the British Empire has changed, and the majority of awards are now given for charity work, and some for contributions to an occupation or position above that to be expected.

Order of the British Empire

I am delighted to say that I was awarded the OBE in June 2012. It was a great honour.

I was surprised when an envelope from the Palace appeared in March of that year, and even more surprised when I opened it. I do remember reading it twice. It said that I must not tell anybody about the honour until it was officially announced, and that I could inform the Palace if I did not wish to receive it. I thought seriously about this question, and about a tenth of a second later reluctantly decided that I would agree to receive it! I will admit that I did tell Vivian, and then realised how difficult it is not to tell anyone else, including my daughters. The official announcement was made on Her Majesty's birthday, and it appeared in the local press that day. The first response was from an overseas friend, who for some peculiar reason must have read through the whole of the honours list that morning. This was followed by various congratulatory letters and emails. We then had to wait for several months before being sent an official invitation, which also allowed three guests to be present at the investiture. One wife and two daughters made it the perfect number.

Then followed the most amazing two days of my life on 18 and 19 October. Vivian organised a visit to the Theatre Royal on the Thursday to see Owaine Arthur in 'One Man. Two Guv'nors'. It was a very late booking and the only seats available were in the front row of the stalls. It was hilarious, and we were very much enjoying it when Owaine came down into the auditorium to recruit two 'helpers', of which I was one. There followed an unscripted dialogue and we then had to carry an object off-stage. Unfortunately we could not lift it, and on turning round discovered Owaine – considerably overweight – standing on it. He then got off and we carted it off into the wings. A few minutes later we were called back on and he asked, 'How did you get on together?' I gave a limp wrist display which was suitably appreciated by the audience. At the end Owaine came down to the stalls and thanked the two of us for our help. By complete chance we met a college friend of Vivian's the next day who had been at the play. She thought that it had all been rehearsed!

On the Friday I was suitably dressed in my morning suit. We had lunch in the Royal Air Force Club with our daughters and son-in-law and 'sin-in-law', and then walked to the Palace. Whilst Vivian, Clare and Tasha were ushered into the hall to listen to a military quartet, I went for a briefing. There I discovered for the first time that I was very luckily to be awarded the medal by Her Majesty herself. We queued up and went in one by one, with our names and reasons for the award being announced, then bowed, had the medal put onto the pin which was already in place, and then exchanged a few words. Her Majesty commented on the fact that my award was for three things – medical services, ornithology and service to the community on the island – and I replied that I was indeed a mixed-up kid. There was a smile and a handshake, and then back into the audience with the medal and its box. Afterwards there were photographs in the courtyard and then home, considerably shattered.

I have not mentioned previously my acting career as it had almost been non-existent and was comprised of three Scout gang shows and two plays at school. So a performance on a London stage and receiving my OBE from Her Majesty in two days was simply incredible.

The award was completely unexpected at the time but in conversations months later with Ken Cunningham, the CEO for many years at Stoke Mandeville Hospital, he told me that I had previously been recommended for an award. And in a conversation with our then Lord Lieutenant, Major General Sir Martin White, I learned that he had recommended to the person (I know not whom) who had organised my application, that contributions other than my medical work should be included, as there are many recommendations for medicine alone and most go no further. I also remember that in 1985 I had been a little upset that I had not been awarded anything after the Bradford Fire as both my friends and colleagues David Sharpe and John Settle received OBEs and the Matron an MBE.

The rules are that one adds the letters post-nominally when the announcement is made, and one can wear the bar or a miniature medal until the investiture, after which the full-size medal is worn on appropriate dress occasions. One advantage of going to military functions and having both St John and Scout uniforms is that I have been able to wear the medal on many occasions. In a conversation with a friend, Geoff Mawson, who received his OBE many years previously, he said that he had never been able to display his, and it had sat in a drawer at his home since the award.

There are two other possible advantages. Firstly the Order has a chapel in St Paul's Cathedral which I can visit at any time, and with no payment. Also a daughter could be married in that chapel. Tasha and Jumbo, however, decided that the Chelsea Registrar's office was more appropriate. I am also entitled to have the College of Arms design a shield for me. Unfortunately this can only be passed down through my non-existent male line. If I am still alive when this changes, as it will, then a shield I will have.

Order of the Most Venerable Order of the Hospital of St John of Jerusalem

My employment and voluntary service with St John are detailed in Chapter 8. One year after my OBE there was another complete surprise when a letter appeared saying that I had been awarded Membership of the Priory of St John. I was invested with this by the Prior almost exactly a year later on 17 October in the Priory Church in East London. The Prior, Admiral Lionel Jervis, had been a colleague of mine at Haslar Hospital and it was therefore also a reunion. Another medal to add to my uniform!

My third and final royal honour was the award of the Officer of St John in 2018. I was unable to attend an investiture in 2019 because of overseas visits and other commitments, and both investitures that I would have attended in 2020 were cancelled because of Covid-19 so it was not until 2021 that I finally received the medal.

Awards

It is easy to define a royal honour, but awards are rather more difficult. My various scholarships and degrees could be considered as awards, and have been partially enunciated earlier. The awards that I have listed here have entailed receiving a medal, a badge or similar.

In 1956 Jamie Rolstone and I were the first two Scouts in our group, the 36th Epping Forest South, to complete the Queen's Scout award for ten years. In the 1950s this had to be done before one's 18th (now 23rd) birthday. We were presented with the badge (which I still wear with pride on my Scout uniform) by the Chief Scout, Lord Rowallan, at Gilwell Park, and we were also invited to Windsor to march past Her Majesty and to attend a service in the Chapel. Soon after obtaining the award, I had interviews both for the industrial scholarship and for selection for the expedition to Arctic Lapland. I still wonder how much effect having a recognised national award on my application forms influenced the results in two very competitive fields.

Many years later in 2011 I was awarded the Scout Wood Badge. This is awarded to a leader when he has completed the mandatory training required, and normally takes one to three years to complete.

At Leeds University I was awarded Half Colours for Sailing in 1960, and Full Colours in 1961. In that same year I was also awarded British Universities Sailing Association (BUSA) Colours. I still have the sweater with BUSA on the front – perhaps appropriately known as a Boozer sweater. At Surrey University, which was then small in numbers, staff often represented the University. I was awarded Colours for Badminton. On my second trip to Cambridge I had become efficient enough on the ice to collect both a Half-Blue and British University Colours for Ice Hockey. And the following year at Oxford – having been suitably attacked in the match by my old colleagues – I got the winning goal and my Oxford Half-Blue.

This was followed by a quiet period of some twenty-five years, and the next awards were for surgery. In 1996 I was appointed the CC Wu Professor by the Chinese University of Hong Kong. As it was an overseas professorship, I did not use the title until recently. Now that overseas titles have become accepted, I am using it. Also in 1996 many of the people who had worked in Sarajevo during the war were invited to return to receive the thanks of the city, and to be presented with a medal. Professor Tony Redmond, the organiser of the whole effort, had done his best for us to be awarded the UN Bosnian Service Medal, and although we had been in greater danger than most of the British troops there at the same time, we were not allowed it as we had not been in uniform. We have since felt that it was particularly unfair, considering that the Ebola medal was allocated to everyone involved – military or civil.

Honours and Awards

In 1999 I was appointed to give the Kannapan Shanmuganathan Oration at the Ganga Hospital in Coimbatore, South India. This remarkable hospital is described in Chapter 9.

In 2006 I was appointed the Wallace Lecturer for that year and received that medal. This is an annual appointment by the British Burn Association to commemorate the contribution to burn care by the recipient, normally over many years, and commemorates the work of A.B. Wallace, the founder of the International Association for Burn Injuries and of the British Association of Plastic Surgeons.

And then in 2007, and out of the blue, although I suspect a cousin of mine may have had some influence, I was made a Fellow of the City of London. Apparently this is uncommon for people who are not members of a livery company. I received the certificate at a ceremony in the Mansion House with my wife and family present, and I can now drive sheep over London Bridge and relieve myself against the rear offside wheel of my carriage – but only within the City.

My final two awards are the Long Service Medal of St John Ambulance, with which I was presented after fifteen years of service in 2013, and the first bar to that medal which I received after a further five years in 2018.

It has, indeed, been an interesting life, and I am proud but somewhat embarrassed at the honours and awards with which I have been presented. I know of many people, including Vivian, who have also done much work in their profession and for charity but have received little or no formal recognition.

Chapter 13

A View of the Changes in Health Care during the last Fifty Years

The year 2022 marks fifty years since I qualified as a doctor, with five more as a medical student before that. Enormous changes, both for good and for bad, have occurred in medicine in that time, both in the world and in Britain. The following are my views of these changes, and refer in particular to surgery in Britain, but also to many other aspects of medicine.

There have been some changes that have been excellent. These include the invention and introduction of Computerised Tomography (CT) and Magnetic Resonance Imaging (MRI) scanners which have both made more accurate and simplified the diagnosis of many diseases. There have been enormous changes in the pharmaceutical industry with new medicines. Much of the surgery for stomach ulcers and for rheumatoid arthritis that I did has now been rendered unnecessary with the introduction of new drugs. On the scientific side, miniaturisation of cameras has also improved diagnosis and also made laparoscopic surgery possible. This has reduced hospital stays and causes smaller scars. And the diagnosis and treatment of some cancers has improved, with at last the possibility of a cure for malignant melanoma where before, if it was missed and not treated by early surgery, there was no further hope.

Another major improvement has been in pre-hospital care with the introduction of trained paramedics. I have slightly mixed feelings about the rigid protocols that the paramedics have to follow at the place of the accident or illness. On rare occasions this can delay urgent transfer to a hospital, which might have resulted in a better outcome.

Two other enormous improvements have been the introduction of air ambulances and a major expansion of the hospice movement. I am utterly convinced that both of these should not be dependent on charitable donations but should come fully within the NHS in the same way that CT and EMI scanners have now done. When these were introduced they were also dependent on donations.

Another change has been the organisation of providing medical and surgical care overseas. I have seen this in the disasters in which I have been involved, and in much of my teaching. The creation of organisations such as Save the Children, Médecins sans Frontières, UK-Med and more recently the UKIETR (United Kingdom International Emergency Trauma Register) have improved the availability of relevant trained staff at short notice. There have also been overseas teaching commitments, often organised by local contacts or for instance in my field by BFIRST (British Foundation for International Reconstructive Surgery and Training) and by UK-Med.

This is an important list of some of the major improvements – but the negative list is in my opinion far longer.

Medical education has changed enormously. Admission to a medical school today is based on 'A' level results, with very few, if any, medical schools now interviewing candidates. I am not convinced that brilliant academic ability is essential, or even a major contributor to being a good doctor. From my own experience, a degree in engineering is considerably more difficult to achieve than a degree in medicine. I would favour candidates who have done something else, for instance being a member of St John Ambulance or worked in a nursing home or a hospital part-time, or as part of a Duke of Edinburgh award. Having doctors or nurses in the family was looked upon favourably as the candidate would have experienced the commitment necessary. Interestingly, I have also found that successful sportsmen and women make good surgeons. Their good hand-to-eye coordination and will to win are both ideals for future surgeons.

There have also been enormous changes in the syllabus. Again from a surgeon's viewpoint, very few medical schools now teach anatomy by human dissection, and from my examining and teaching over the last few years I sometimes wonder if they teach anatomy at all! There has also been a huge increase in the number of students in nearly all medical schools, and I was lucky to have only twenty-six students in my year in Oxford, compared to the larger numbers in London hospitals to which went many of my undergraduate friends. I will admit that psychology and how to talk to patients are now widely taught – but somehow with our small numbers we picked this up as we went along – although my wife might disagree.

One definite loss has been that of the student locum appointments that existed when I was a student. These were incredibly useful as an introduction to being a junior doctor with a controlled back-up.

A View of the Changes in Health Care during the last Fifty Years

On qualifying, my vintage spent one year as a house officer and then normally two years as a senior house officer (SHO) in a variety of subjects. These posts did not need a formal interview panel and, as mine were, had sometimes been arranged during student times or house officer posts. After the SHO posts, and having decided what specialty one wished to pursue, one started looking for a formal registrar post in that specialty. These were competitive and required a formal interview. There could be fifty or a hundred applicants for a single post. The application was submitted with a CV, and references from the present or previous employers. These were sometimes supplemented by recommendations on the telephone. It was expected that additional qualifications, research papers, etc., were also submitted. A short list of normally six was made and they were called for interview. One great advantage of that system, particularly in surgery, was that an estimate of surgical ability could be garnered from the telephone and personal comments and references from the people for whom a candidate had worked, which of course is not measurable by interview. Now, telephone conversations are banned and the references are not considered until the decision is made. I know of several instances where inappropriate appointments have been made of candidates who had the knowledge and qualifications, and gave an excellent interview – but could not operate. It is now extremely difficult to curtail an appointment. I have sat on several appeal committees concerning this – but again, how does one measure operative ability outside the operating theatre?

The registrar post would last up to two years, and this could be lengthened by mutual agreement. The next stage was a senior registrar post, which was four years of formal training, and could include research or travel time, and extend to six years. This was wholly competitive, and people who were not successful might be advised to consider another specialty. And then, if all had been satisfactory, there was the final competitive interview for a consultant. This would be, if all went well, for the remainder of one's working life up to 65 years old. The total length of time between qualifying and a consultant post depended very much on the specialty. Anaesthetics was probably the shortest at a minimum of seven years. I took just under thirteen years and was the second most rapid in plastic surgery at the time.

In 2005 the whole system changed. The post of house officer (now known as a Foundation Doctor) became two years, and then there was one competitive interview to obtain a junior recognised training post. The short list for interview had to be made without any communication with previous employers, and no reference could be read until an appointment had been made. The disadvantages to the new system are obvious. Firstly, a decision concerning one's future career has to be made in the second year without the option of trying other specialties to enable a more definitive choice of career. Secondly, the one interview is very early after registration and the short listing is done purely on the CV, with no other input. Thirdly, the references could only be of use if there was a definite reason for disbarring the candidate who was successful at interview, for example for criminal misbehaviour. But the real problem was the inability to assess the surgical ability of a prospective surgeon. In each year of the training programme a report is made on the candidate, and if they have proved unsatisfactory, they can in theory be thrown off the programme. But this may be appealed, and I sat on several appeal committees which were difficult and rarely satisfactory. Under the old system, the candidate was simply not promoted.

There is also less incentive to get involved in a research project. Under the old system the interviews to registrar and senior registrar positions were more likely to be successful if the junior had published one or more research papers. Many then did no further research in their careers, but others became involved. I remember one junior with whom I worked in Bradford, who was not progressing up the ladder. After the Bradford Fire, and other projects in which I involved him, he suddenly started writing and publishing, went rapidly up the ladder and is still publishing.

I can see only one advantage for the doctor from this change, and that was not absolute, in that one generally only needs to buy one house now as a formal trainee, as the training is in one region.

The system is clearly not working. In one recent report 37 per cent of people finishing their foundation years left the NHS, either to work overseas or to change careers completely. In my time as a junior doctor I would work either one night and weekend in two or one in three on call – as well as all the hours of each weekday. Dependent on the rota, this would be a total of 114 or 89 hours a week, and this would increase to cover the holiday time of the other person(s) in the rota. In only one locum post was my commitment one in one on call: 168 hours a week. Some of this time one could be asleep. Or, as progression up the ranks occurred, at home. But long-range bleeps and mobile phones did not exist and one was severely limited as to what one could do.

The major change that happened in 1993 was the introduction of the EU working time directive. Junior doctors were no longer allowed to work more than 48 hours per week on average, and had to have designated rest times after a night on call. The rules laid down by the British Government enabled consultants, but not junior doctors, to opt out of this commitment if they wished. The consequences of this were very obvious and twofold. There had to be an enormous increase in the numbers of junior doctors, and each received far less experience in their training. Some hospitals took this to mad levels and banned a junior staying in the hospital in their own time to watch the finish of a clinic or an operation, saying that they were not insured. When I joined Stoke Mandeville in 1985 there were seven of us in the department. When I left in 2001 there were nineteen in the department, and we had lost some of our catchment area.

The situation for training was made even worse by a theoretical shortening of the time from qualifying to consultant. Analysis by the Royal College of Surgeons showed a reduction in operating hours' experience by as much as 75 per cent. In one report some years ago it stated that 12 per cent of newly appointed consultant surgeons were suspended for further training within the first year of appointment. These are horrifying figures, and responsible were the European working time directive and the changes in training introduced in 2005. Will Brexit be able to reverse the situation? I sincerely hope so. When I am teaching and talking to junior doctors, certainly amongst surgeons there is a strong wish for this reversal to happen – at least in part – so that their operative experience and skill can be increased.

Another very valuable aspect of the old system, particularly in clinical subjects, was that the care of the patient was in firms. A firm consisted of one to three consultants and a selection of junior trainees who would remain as a group for weeks or months. This meant that 24-hour care was always being done by someone who knew the background of every patient who was being looked after by a firm. Now the junior being called in the middle of the night will probably not have seen the patient before, and also may not have had a handover before coming on duty. Without a doubt this is detrimental to patient care.

Other changes that have happened, again to a large extent caused by the above developments, are that there has been an increase in consultant numbers and more specialisation within surgical specialties. I had two main specialties and two minor specialties. Among new consultants now more than one is a rarity. This is said not to be a disadvantage, but if a multiply injured patient is admitted, the old wider base of experience was often essential for the best result.

Not related to the EU directive, there have been six changes following government policies within my timescale as a consultant.

Firstly, under Mrs Thatcher's government it was decided that the cost of all treatment would be calculated. This required a large increase in management personnel. When I joined Stoke Mandeville in 1985 there were three managers within the hospital. When I left in 2001 there were three corridors full of them! I have never seen any report saying that money was saved, and I very much suspect that the cost of collecting the information was greater than any saving.

The second change that occurred over a period lasting several years was a large decrease in the number of hospital beds available. My own plastic surgery and burn unit reduced from eighty beds to approximately forty beds. This was partially justified as patients were staying in for shorter times, but was not justified by the management requirement in line with the NHS directive for the bed occupancy to be 100 per cent. This has resulted in patients regularly waiting in corridors for a bed. One other consequence for surgical patients has been a very large increase of re-admissions following the early discharge times required. A final problem has been that patients who require specialised nursing are often 'boarded' on a ward away from the specialised nursing that is required, to the discomfort of patients and nurses. The 100 per cent occupancy directive on occasions worked during the summer months, but not in the winter. The severity of the problem became even more obvious during the Covid-19 pandemic. There are insufficient beds now for the acute patients, and the enormous rise in patients waiting for surgery, often urgent operations, is increasing all the time. We have almost the lowest percentage of hospital beds for the population of any country in Europe.

A third change that has occurred is that after 5.00pm only an emergency with possible loss of life or limb may go to theatre. In the past, most emergency surgery, including less severe problems, would be operated on at night. This was excellent for junior doctor training, and also meant that the booked admissions for the following day were not cancelled at short notice.

The fourth even more recent change, which was just happening in 2001, was that no consultant had a waiting list of their own, and the waiting list was shared within the department. This is an absolute disaster as each consultant had one or more specialties and would be unable to operate safely or properly on a patient with a different sub-specialty problem.

A View of the Changes in Health Care during the last Fifty Years

The fifth change has been the loss of personal secretaries in many hospitals, and with the typing now sometimes being done overseas. Having my secretary in the clinic, and able to do shorthand, meant that I saw approximately double the number of patients in each clinic than would otherwise have been possible.

Finally, and probably the biggest disaster of all, was the decision under Tony Blair's government to stop the 24-hour cover of their patients by general practitioners in 1996, in return for a small decrease in their salaries. My wife was a GP at that time in a small country practice where she and her practice partner knew their patients. If Mrs Smith phoned up at two o'clock in the morning with severe chest pain, the advice was to take an aspirin and come to the surgery the next day. This was only possible because they knew Mrs Smith, who for the past ten years had phoned up at regular intervals with the same problem, and really only wanted a chat. A GP covering after hours would not know Mrs Smith, and with that story an urgent 999 ambulance would have to be sent.

When the change occurred, 24-hour cover was sometimes organised locally, but less so in London and other large cities, and overseas doctors would fly to Britain to do weekend cover and to earn money. Many of these doctors spoke little English. My wife did this cover for some time, but instead of looking after 5,000 patients would be on call for 70,000 or more patients of whom she had no prior knowledge. She hated this so much that she retired early, as did many other GPs. After my wife's and my time in the NHS this changed again, with a new GP contract in 2004. However, the number of people with a variety of problems now walking into casualty (Accident and Emergency) departments where they are guaranteed to be seen is very large and has completely changed how such departments now work. The waiting times to be seen in A&E increased, and in 2001 a maximum limit of 4 hours was put on this time, and if the hospital failed then it was fined. This could mean that unnecessary patients were admitted or were discharged before they had been fully evaluated. Theoretically perhaps it was good idea, but in practice it is another disaster.

There have also been negative changes to the nursing profession. The famous author, raconteur and surgeon Professor Harold Ellis was the principal guest speaker at a joint meeting of the British and American Hand Societies some years ago in Cambridge. His speech started, '1948 was a very important year for medicine in this country. The Health Service was founded, and I qualified.' He then went on to describe the changes that had occurred in nursing care, finishing up with, 'And all these changes have been to the detriment of nursing care.' The British surgeons present all cheered, and very obviously agreed with his comments. The Americans looked baffled.

In my fifty years nursing has indeed changed. The training of State Enrolled Nurses (SENs) was abandoned in 1989. Although of a lower academic standard, the SENs were very often excellent hands-on nurses. Around that time Project 2000 began to be implemented as the nursing organisations thought that with the increasing complexity of medicine, a higher academic level was required. Most of the doctors and a lot of the nurses disagreed with this, but by 2009 all new nurses had to have a degree. Much of the basic nursing care that was done by the SENs was taken over by nursing assistants. Although many of these are excellent, they have considerably less training than the two years of the SENs. They also earn less.

So now we have degree-level nurses with less training in basic nursing, and less well qualified nursing assistants. I have yet to see any evidence that this has improved the nursing care of our patients, and it has led to considerable disquiet from many people. And there is still a shortage of nurses, although one of the very few good things about Covid-19 has been an increase in people wanting a career in nursing.

There have been changes in the patients as well. Obesity has become more common and has even led to the development of the new specialty of bariatric surgery. Obesity also leads to greater wear on joints, and therefore an increase in demand for joint replacements. Diabetes has also increased, and its treatment adds to the demands on the NHS. Other problems are an increase in psychiatric cases, and also in family breakdowns, both of which again demand more care and more money. And for the first time for generations, life expectancy in Britain is decreasing.

My final thoughts in this chapter involve what I see as the problems for the future. Medically these must include antibiotic resistance. There are already warnings about this, and the chances of major problems are being exacerbated by the widespread misuse of antibiotics particularly in many overseas countries, and also by their use in farming and agriculture, etc.

I am much more hopeful about pandemics. We have learned a lot during the present Covid-19 pandemic. Anti-viral vaccines have been a great success, and the use of live wild animal markets and bush-meat has reduced, and will I think reduce further. One remaining problem is the rate of initial spread because of air travel and movements between countries.

A View of the Changes in Health Care during the last Fifty Years

Climate change is on everyone's lips. Yes, it is happening, and we know to some extent why, and how it can be reduced. It is to be hoped that all countries, and especially the richer nations who are more responsible for the change, will do what is needed. If not, then increasing food and water shortages worldwide will inevitably lead to wars.

The one thing that everybody is not talking about, because it is politically and religiously difficult, is that there are too many people on this planet, and the numbers in many countries are still rapidly increasing. The problem has been to a large degree of our own making, with colonisation and then improvements in medical care. Since the industrial revolution the number of children born and surviving infancy has increased enormously, and the average age of death has also almost doubled. There have been catastrophes, such as the bubonic plague (the Black Death), which killed 20 per cent of the population of Europe, and the 1918 flu epidemic, when the death rate was 3 per cent. It was far worse in South America, where more than 90 per cent were killed when smallpox was brought in by colonists. But as can be seen by the response to Covid-19, these mortality figures are much reduced by modern medical developments in prevention and treatment.

China is, I believe, the only country that has tried to reduce its population with the one-child policy, but the preponderance of males born and surviving has made this unacceptable. One Hong Kong friend of mine has two sons. I asked him whether he would have been happy had they been girls. His reply was that he would not have been upset, but his parents would have wanted them to have another child to try to get a male to carry on the family line. And that explains the failure of the one-child policy.

From recent research reports, it seems possible that nature is curing the problem itself. There has been a marked decrease in the numbers of babies born, particularly in western nations over the past thirty years. This has no doubt several causes, but one proven cause is the reduction in viable sperm produced by males, not only in western nations but also in China, India and Africa. The combination of increasing population, which is still occurring, and climate change will lead to the loss of the beauty and biodiversity of our world as more food has to be grown to feed the expanding population. The only hopes for the near future are education and the acceptance of birth control measures.

This is a very depressing outlook for our children and even more so for our grandchildren. I cannot see the answers to this problem, but somehow politicians and religious leaders must change the present situation, and rapidly, or the population will continue to grow, at least in the short and medium terms, and so will hunger, mass migration, global warming and the break-up of civilisations.

Summary

It has been for me a remarkable eighty-three years. For somebody who started life as the only child of a couple who were to be divorced when I was about 4 or 5, and then to be seriously ill to the extent that I did not start school until I was nearly 8, to finish up living in a fourteenth-century Manor House with my own nature reserve that I have created around it, and with a large number of letters after my name, including the OBE and the OStJ, is unusual. I was born with three major advantages: firstly, I was intelligent, with a measured IQ at Cambridge of 164. Secondly, I had a near-photographic memory. I could play bridge for twelve hours and the next day tell you every card played by every player. I wish that I could still do it! And thirdly, and I am not sure if this was born into me or developed by me, I have always believed in having a go at doing something different or unusual, whenever the chance was offered to me.

Much of my early life and my survival depended on my mother's remarkable efforts. She had had virtually no formal education, but was extremely intelligent herself – she could do the *Daily Telegraph* cryptic crossword in 15 minutes, which was her norm unless it was indeed a bad day. And with almost no money in the family, she allowed me to do what was possible, and she was almost certainly the person who taught me to read, write and do arithmetic before my late start at school. She gave up almost everything, but unfortunately not her smoking, and this was the major cause of her chronic ill-health, her inability to take part in any active pastimes and her eventual death.

I was lucky in that scholarships were on offer, and of these I took full advantage. Without those scholarships who knows where I would now be. Much as I enjoyed my engineering intellectually, and still do, the job of management that went with it I found abhorrent. Luckily I was then unmarried, and the only person who suffered financially when I changed career from engineering to medicine was me. As my medical career progressed, opportunities to go to Africa and America came along, and partly through my efforts, and partly through luck and scholarships, I was able to take full advantage of these. The posts that I held during my training, and the way in which some of these posts were obtained, were again almost, but not quite, pure luck. I remember at my first surgical conference a

A View of the Changes in Health Care during the last Fifty Years

presentation by Geoffrey Page. A pilot who had been shot down in the Second World War, he was treated by Sir Archibald McIndoe at East Grinstead. He was also a founder of the Guinea Pig Club, and later the President after McIndoe's death. He inspired me to work in burns, which is not the most popular specialty. I had found the two surgical loves of my life, the treatment of burns and hand surgery, from these posts. They are an interesting combination in that burn surgery is simple, but the patients can be medically extremely challenging, but in hand surgery the real challenge is in surgical ability.

And then, just before starting my consultant career, the Bradford Fire occurred on 11 May 1985. My involvement with this, and the two lecture tours that followed afterwards to Australia and to South Africa, established me on the international lecture circuit and of this I have taken very full advantage over the whole of my consultant career.

My early life as an engineer and my medical training to consultant level has been more fully described in *Scholarship Boy to Engineer, Plastic Surgeon and Sportsman* which has been recently published.

I have, of course, had disappointments in my life: failing the medical to fly with the Royal Air Force, in sport, where I failed in the Olympic sailing trials in 1971 – having placed second all year, we only came fifth. And my first engagement, which ended when Moira decided that she could not take on the responsibility of marriage, and in fact she never did. But when I met and married Vivian, my wife of fifty years, this disappointment became much less.

During my life I have met a remarkable number of well known people, including Her Majesty and Winston Churchill.

I am still involved both in teaching – surgeons, bird ringers and sailors – and am also President of 'Restore – Burn and Wound Research' and of St John Ambulance on the Isle of Wight. I am still involved in Scouting as the Vice President of the Scout Association on the island, and in natural history as Chairman of the Isle of Wight Bird-Ringing Group and of the Publications Committee of the Isle of Wight Natural History and Archaeological Society. I have now reduced my skiing and sailing, but active reconstruction continues with a large amount of work around the manor house and the reserve.

And more and more I believe in the old adage: Sudden death is nature's way of telling one to slow down.

References

Desai, Sanu N., *Neonatal Surgery of the Cleft Lip* (World Scientific Publishing Co., 1998).

Fletcher, Martin, *Fifty-six: The Story of the Bradford Fire* (2015).

Malcolm, Noel, *Bosnia. A Short History* (Macmillan, 1997).

Malcolm, Noel, *Kosovo. A Short History* (Macmillan, 1997).

Page, Geoffrey, *Tale of a Guinea Pig* (Pelham Books, 1981).

Roberts, Anthony, *Scholarship Boy to Engineer, Plastic Surgeon and Sportsman* (Matador, 2022).

Silver, John R., 'A History of Stoke Mandeville Hospital and the National Spinal Injuries Centre', *Journal of the Royal College of Physicians, Edinburgh*, 2019, 49:328–3.

Watkins, Syd, *Life at the Limit* (Macmillan, 1997).

References

Index

Abu Dhabi, UAE, 144
Accident Service, Oxford, 35, 178
Acid Survivors Foundation Hospital, Bangladesh, 146
Adie, Kate, CBE, BBC, 69, 90, 161
Advanced Trauma Life Support (ATLS) course, 108, 110, 153
Ahmedabad, Gujerat, India, 136
Ainslie, Sir Ben, 119
Akrotiri, Cyprus, 61
Alexander, Lord, 39
Alexander of Weedon, Lady, 37
Andrews, Dr Francis, 25
Angus, Dr Jim, 6
Armenia, 99, 101
Arthur, Owain, Actor, 181
Association of Anaesthetists, 75
Aston Martin, 105
Atkinson Morley Neurology Hospital, 109
Attwood, Sqn Ldr Tony, 13
Austin Hospital, Melbourne, 6
Australia, x, 1, 72, 132
Australian Flying Doctor Service, 9
Aylesbury, Buckinghamshire, 15
Azerbaijan, 20, 99, 101, 144

Bahrami, Mansour, Tennis player, 121
Bailey, Bruce, 13, 15, 26, 31, 37, 40, 177
Baillie, Fiona, 18
Baku, Azerbaijan, 100
Bancroft's School, ix, 43
Band, George, OBE, 119
Bangladesh, 146
Bannerjee, Sonia, 6
Banwell, Paul, 42

Barclay, Tom, 16, 31, 36, 68, 131
Barnett, Robert, British Ambassador, 93
Battle Hospital, Reading, 15, 25, 178
Beer, Dr Tim, 26
Bell, Derek, MBE, Le Mans winner, 110
Bell, John, American racing driver, 110
Bellingham, Sqn Ldr Don, 14
Bellingham, Lynda, 14
Bennett, Lt Col. Nicholas, 58
Benson, Sister Jacky, 32, 88
Bilwani, Dr P.K., India, 136
Bird banding/ringing, 12, 197
Birmingham Accident Hospital, 19, 21, 35, 41, 51, 66, 131, 147, 152, 173
Black Arrows Aerobatic Team, 47
Blair, Sir Anthony, 193
Bosnia, 21, 56, 87, 98, 131
Botswana, 142
Botting, Dr Jonathan, 112
Bowen, Vaughan, 3
Bradford, vii, 6, 36, 190
Bradford Football Stadium Fire, x, 14, 36, 51, 66, 90, 158, 183
Bradford Royal Infirmary, 67
Brands Hatch Motor Racing Circuit, 109
Branson, Sir Richard, 37
Brathay Foundation, Faeroes, 148
British Army Training Unit, Suffield (BATUS), Canada, 63
British Association of Plastic Surgeons, 12, 75, 87
British Burn Association, 28, 147
British Military Surgical Society, 63, 131, 147
British Orthopaedic Association, 75
British Racing Drivers Club, 107

British Schools Exploring Society, 147
British Standards Institute, 28
Brown, Air Commodore Ronnie, 54, 59
Brown, Dr Raymond, 22
Brunei, 1
Buckingham, Buckinghamshire, 22
Buckingham Hospital, 25, 27
Buckingham Palace, 125
Budny, Peter, 17
Bugatti, 105
Bunsell, Dr Richard, 16, 20, 21, 88, 92, 101, 120, 176
Burge, Dr Susan, 25
Burns and Plastics Unit SMH, viii, 36
Button, Jenson, MBE, 111

C C Wu Professorship, Hong Kong, 134, 184
Cairns, Queensland, Australia, 9
Cairo, 140
Cambodia, 147
Cambridge, x
Campbell, Gavin, 37, 158
Campbell, Surgeon Captain James, 60
Cape York Peninsula, 9
Carrington, Lord, 40
Catherine, secretary, 25
Cavendish Laboratory, Cambridge, 151
Cebu University, Philippines, 145
Chapman, Peter, 39, 113
Cheltenham General Hospital, 105
Chen, Hung-Chi, 3
Chengdu, Sichuan, China, 135
Chiltern Hospital, Great Missenden, 31
Chinese University of Hong Kong, 133, 184
Christ Church, Oxford, 152
Christie, Brian, 16
Churchill, Sir Winston, viii, 197
Clare College, Cambridge, 151
Clarke, Maria, 22, 88
Clinton, President Bill, 21
Cockin, John, 35
Collins, Sir Alan KCVO and Lady Ann, Philippines, 134, 145, 160

Colquhoun, Mr and Mrs, Medical Support Romania, 145
Cooke, Jan, 20
Covid-19, ix, 192, 194
Coy's Historic Car Festival, 106
Cranston, Dr David, F1, 108
Crockett, David, 36, 68
Cross, Maj. Randall, MBE, 126
Crown Prosecution Service, 164
Cunningham, Ken, vii, 29, 182
Currie, Edwina, MP, 29

Daimler V8 sports car, 112
Daring, HMS, 63
Das, Dr Suman, 3
Deere, Group Captain Al, 46
Desai, Sanu, 13, 16, 31, 38
Dettori, Frankie, 108
Dhaka University Hospital, Bangladesh, 145
Dhekelia, Cyprus, 61
Diamond, Anne, ITV, 70
Dickinson, John, 18
Doll, Prof. Sir Richard, 37, 40
Dominican Republic, 75, 79
Dominie, De Havilland, 48
Donington Motor Racing Circuit, 113
Doyle, Carol, 32
Dunkin, Chris, 42
Dupuytren's Disease, 70

Eaglemont, Victoria, 11
Ecclestone, Bernie, 107
Egypt, 139
Ejeskar, Dr Arvid, 130
El Sawy, Gen. Mohammed, Cairo, 140
Eldolify, Prof. General Ezz, 139
Elefsina Oil Refinery, Athens, 72
Ellis, Prof. Harold, CBE, 193
European Union Working Hours Directive, 190
Everett, Bill, 31

Falkland Islands, 149
Feenan, Maj. Paul, 63
Fellow of the City of London, 185

Index

Fennell, Sir Desmond, 37, 40
Ferrari, 107
Festival of Speed, Goodwood, 109
Fire Safe Cigarette Campaign, 28
Fort Blockhouse, Royal Navy, 58
Fowler, Baron Norman, Kt, PC, 119
Fox, Sister Susan, 20, 72
Frankel, Dr Hans, 24

Galsworthy, Sir Anthony and Lady Jan, 133
Ganga Hospital, Coimbatore, Tamil Nadu, 137, 185
Gardner, Brian, 24
General Medical Council (GMC), 23
Gill, Dr Kate, Motor Racing, 112
Gillett, Dr Paul, 22
Gloucester, The Duke and Duchess of, 119, 124
Go Karting, 108
Goddard, Anthony, Racing Driver, 112
Golden bower birds, 11
Goodwood Motor Racing Circuit, 109
Gordina, Dr Marko, 18
Graham, Lord Calum, 40
Grogono, James, 27
Guinea Pig Club, 197
Gulf of Carpentaria, 10
Gulf Wars, 51, 54, 63, 87
Gunn, Rodney, 56
Gupta, Prof. Malti, India, 137
Guttmann, Sir Ludwig, 15, 23

Hadassah Hospital, Jerusalem, 85, 138
Haiti, 74
Hamilton, Sir Lewis, F1 champion, 111
Harris, Prof., Oxford, 39
Hartwell, Lord, 40
Haseley Manor, Isle of Wight, 118, 126, 196
Hay, Brenner, 88
Heartline Charity, USA, 76
Heath, Gordon, 50
Heidelberg Repatriation Hospital, 3
Heimbach, Dr David, Seattle, 138
Helmia Military Hospital, Cairo, 140

Henderson, Nigel, Surgeon, 120
Hercules Aeroplane, C130, 88, 95
Herndon, Dr David, USA, 133
Heywood, Tony, 17, 24
High Wycombe Hospital, 25, 27
Higham, Prof. Charles, ONZM, 119
Hiles, Ronald, OBE, 146
Hill, Alison, 21
Hill, Phil, F1 Champion, 108
HIV and AIDS, 143
Holiday Inn, Sarajevo, 89, 98
Hong Kong, 73, 131
Honorary Civilian Consultant RAF, 56
Hormbrey, Liz, 42
Horn, Sister Diana, 20
Horwood and James, Solicitors, 38
Houses of Parliament, 29
Hughes, Dr Amy, MBE, 79
Hugh-Smith, Sir Andrew, 38
Hujic, Dr, Sarajevo, 91, 96
Hunt, Michael, 88
Hweidi, Prof. Sobhi, 141

Inchcape, The Earl of, 37, 40
India, 136
Internally Displaced Persons (IDPs), 99
International Society for Burn Injuries, 28, 72, 132, 136, 139
International Society of Hand Surgeons, 138
Isle of Wight, 58, 109, 115, 118, 197
Ismaeli, Col. Muri, 61

Jackson, Douglas, 28, 41, 131, 136
Jackson, Michael, Pop singer, 161
Jackson, Moya, British Council, Philippines, 145
Jaipur, Rajasthan, India, 137
Japan, 139
Jenkins, Dr Andrew, 3
Jenkins, Vice Admiral Ian, 56
Jenner, David, 3
Jervis, Rear Admiral Lionel, 60, 183
Jesus College, Cambridge, 175
John Radcliffe Hospital, Oxford, 27, 61
Johnson, Boris, PM, 125

Jones, Sister Adele, 20
Jones, Alan, F1 champion, 111

Kearton, Lord, 40
Kent, The Duke of, 25, 40, 107, 119, 126, 144
Kilner, Prof. T. Pomfret, 15
King, Prof. Walter, Hong Kong, 74, 133, 135
Kinnock, Neil and Glenys, 70
Kinvig, John and Margaret, South Africa, 149
Kirkham, Alyson, 32
Knesevic, Dr Zjelka, Sarajevo, 93, 98
Kosovo, Kosovans, 101, 131
Kurtagic, Nadja and Effe, 94, 97

Lamont, Dr Alastair, Botswana, 143
Le Mans 24hr Race, 106, 110
Leeds, Yorkshire, 14
Leggatt, Alan, cousin, 49
Leonard Cheshire Dept of Conflict Recovery, 100
Li, Prof. Arthur, GBM, Hong Kong, 133
Liu, Alison, Hong Kong, 132
Livingstone, Ken, MP, 29
Ljubljana, Yugoslavia, 18
Llewellyn Jones, Jeremy, BBC producer, 88
Lochaitis, Dr, Greece, 72
Lockerbie, 65
London, Peter, 51
Longmoor Farm, Aston Abbotts, 14
Lords Cricket Ground, 122
Lotus Cars, 109
Lourie, Prof. John, 27
Loyn, Dr Richard, 12
Lymphodaemia, 5, 36
Lynn, Dame Vera, 125

Maadi Military Hospital, Cairo, 140
McElroy, Bernie, 106
McGrouther, Prof. Gus, 39, 41, 144
McIndoe, Sir Archibald, 36, 197
McKay, Nurse Sue, 5
McLeod, Allan, 3

Mace, Martin, 16
Machlachan, Dr Allan, 14
Magdalen College, Oxford, 152
Maier, Penny, 32
Malaysia, 1
Malcolm, Noel, Author, 98
Malignant melanoma, 15
Maltman's Green Preparatory School, 14
Mansell, Nigel, CBE 39
March, Earl of (Duke of Richmond), 109, 111
Maridi, South Sudan, 82
Mason, Prof. Sir Ronald, 37, 40
Matthews, John, Isle of Wight, 166
Matthews, Richard, 13
Maxwell, Robert, 71
May, P.B.H., Cricketer 122
Maybe Airlines, 88, 96
Médecins San Frontières (MSF), 82, 96, 150, 188
Medical Defence Union (MDU), 161
Medical Disasters, 65
Melbourne, Australia, 1, 2, 36
Menzies, Lt Gen. Bob, CB, OBE, 117
MERLIN, Medical Emergency Relief International, 75
Merriweather, Rev. Dr Alfred, CBE, 143
Meteor Aeroplanes, 48
Methodist Ladies College, 11
Microsurgery, 4, 36, 98
Military (Swiss Cheese) Hospital, Sarajevo, 90
Miller, Col., USAF, 52
Milton Keynes Hospital, 25, 27, 56
Minton, Dr Clive and Pat, 1
Miscampbell, Gillian, 13, 29, 37
Moberg, Dr Eric, Sweden, 130
Moffat, Rev. Dr Howard and Fiona, 142
Mohammed, Dr, Sarajevo, 90
Moore, William, 1
Morgans, Air Commodore Bryan, 59
Morley, Air Vice Marshal, 54
Morrison, Tom and Fi, 101
Morrison, Wayne, 2
Moscow, 142
Moss, Sir Stirling, 109, 111

Index

Mossad, Dr, 67
Mount Vernon Hospital, 2, 72
Mubarak, Suzanne, Egypt, 141

Nagorno-Karabakh, 99, 101
Nakas, Dr, Sarajevo, 91
National Health Service (NHS), 30, 162, 175, 187
National Service, 49
National Spinal Injuries Unit, viii, 23, 30
Navein, Col. John, 57, 96
Naylor, James, 40
Neal, Liz, 25
Newcastle, 35
Newing, Dr Richard, 2
Newman, John, MBE, SJA, 117
Newnham College, Cambridge, 151
Nicholson, Amanda, 39
Nightingale, Dr Geraldine, 5
Noone, Dr Cathy, 22
Northampton General Hospital, 15, 25, 107
Not Forgotten Association, 125
Nuseibeh, Dr Isaac, 24

O'Brien, Bernard, 1, 5, 31
O'Brien Institute, 2
Old House, The, Whitchurch, 32
One Man, Two Guv'nors, Theatre Royal, 181
Order of the British Empire, xi, 181
Order of St John, xi, 115, 127, 183
Ovid, 86, 103
Oxford Region Burn Unit, 13, 15, 19, 51

Page, Geoffrey, RAF, 197, 199
Pandya, Wg Co. Ankur, 58
Papadopoulos, Dr Orthon, 3
Papini, Raymond, 75
Papua New Guinea, 10, 139
Paralympics, 24
Parkinson's Disease, 15
Parotid tumours, 16
Peking (Beijing), 135
Philippines, 1, 63, 81, 145
Pinderfield's Hospital, Wakefield, 69

Pleat, Jonathan, 41
Ponting, Jayne, 26
Popplewell Enquiry, 72
Port au Prince, 74
Post Traumatic Stress Disorder (PTSD), 71
Prescott Hill Climb, 105, 113
Pribaz, Dr Julian, 13
Prince Charles, 70
Princess Marina Hospital, Botswana, 143
Princess Mary's Hospital, RAF Akrotiri, 54, 61
Pristina, Kosovo, 101
Pruitt, Col. Basil, 73

Queen Alexandra's Hospital, Cosham, 59
Queen Elizabeth Hospital, Birmingham, 61
Queen Elizabeth II, 125, 181, 182
Queen Victoria Hospital, East Grinstead, 36, 197

Rainford, Air Commodore David, 54
Rank, Sir Benjamin, 2
Rantzen, Dame Esther, 29, 159
Ratcliffe, Rob, 72
Red Cross, 117, 125
Red Cross Children's Hospital, Cape Town, 132
Redmond, Prof. Tony, OBE, 79, 82, 87, 92, 184
Reed, Clive, 3
Regan, Padraic, 17
Reid, William, Glasgow, 155
Research Trust, 32, 37
Restore – Burn and Wound Research, 38
Retinitis pigmentosa, 2
Revival Meeting, Goodwood, 109
Rheumatoid Arthritis, 26
Rider, Steve, F1 commentator, 111
Roberts, Clare, 14
Roberts, Dr Ian, F1, 108
Roberts, Natasha, 11, 14
Roberts, Dr Vivian, ix, 9, 14, 97, 102, 118, 126, 129, 140, 143, 181, 185, 197
Rode, Prof. Hans, South Africa, 132

Romania, 145
Rothschild, Sir Evelyn, 38
Royal Air Force, 25, 43, 46, 51, 56, 88, 95, 123, 170, 197
Royal Air Force Club, 59, 117, 182
Royal Australasian College of Surgeons, 8
Royal Australian Air Force, 3
Royal Canadian Air Force, 56, 88
Royal College of Physicians, 24, 26
Royal College of Surgeons, 24, 28, 117, 137, 153, 155, 191
Royal College of Surgeons of Glasgow, 144, 155
Royal Hospital, Haslar, 58, 64
Royal Melbourne Hospital, 2, 6
Royal Navy, 51
Royal Protection Group, xi, 118, 124
Royal Society, The, 37, 40
Royal Society of Medicine, 40, 71
Russia, 142
Ryan, Prof. Col. Jim, 100

Sabapathy, Dr Raja, 137
St Catharine's College, Cambridge, x, 94, 151
St Edmund Hall, Oxford, 151
St John Ambulance, 60, 83, 110, 115, 158, 185, 188, 197
St Luke's Hospital, Bradford, 68
St Mary's Hospital, Isle of Wight, 83
St Mary's Hospital, London, 123
St Mary's Military Hospital, RAF Halton, 25, 54
St Petersburg, Russia, 142
St Vincent's Hospital, 1, 13
Salmon, Dr Michael, 30
Sarajevo, 56, 87, 88, 96, 101, 130, 160, 184
Save the Children (SAVE), 83, 188
Savile, Sir James (Jimmy), 30
Sawyer, Oliver, 84
Saxon Clinic, Milton Keynes, 32
Scerri, Group Captain Godwin, 53, 57
Scholarship Boy to Engineer, Plastic Surgeon and Sportsman, x
Schumacher, Michael, 107

Schwarzenegger, Arnold, 108
Scott, Mark, 17
Scottish Mission Hospital, Molepolole, 143
Secker-Walker, David, 49
Second World War, 20, 30, 86
Serbia, Serbs, 89, 93, 98, 103
Settle, Dr John, OBE, 69, 183
Sharpe, David, OBE, 67, 183
Shelter Boxes, 77
Siege Doctors, BBC4 Documentary series, 93, 160
Silver, Dr John, 24
Silverstone Motor Racing Track, 29, 106, 110
Simmonds, Nancy, 20
Simson, Jay and Annie 110, 113
Smallwood, Chris, 25
Smith, Dr Gary, F1, 111
Smith and Nephew Foundation, 71, 97
South Africa, 132
South Sudan, 82, 150
Southern Africa, Plastic and Reconstructive Surgeons of, 132
Special Air Service (SAS), 51, 56, 57, 95, 171
Srebrenica, 95
Srpska, 98
Stanley, Prof. John, 26
Stewart, Sir Jackie, 107
Stoke Mandeville Hospital, viii, x, 13, 19, 31, 36, 40, 51, 61, 72, 88, 115, 129, 133, 139, 153, 158, 163, 191
Sumeray, Caroline, Isle of Wight, 166
Sun Yat Sen, Dr, China, 134
Surtees, John, CBE, 39, 107, 111
Sydney, Australia, 8

Tacloban, Philippines, 81
Tawny Frogmouth, 5
Taylor, Andrew, 6
Teddy, Peter, 35
Thatcher, Margaret, PM, and Denis, 70, 192
That's Life, 29, 37, 158
Three Shires Hospital, Northampton, 32

Index

Thruxton Motor Racing Circuit, 109, 113
Titchmarsh, Alan, MBE, 119
Tomkins, Sir Edward, 37, 40
Trinity Hall, Cambridge, 151
Tudway, Dr Andrew, 18
Twickenham Rugby Ground, 119
Tyler, Michael, 17, 40, 41

UK Med, 79, 87, 188
United Kingdom International
 Emergency Relief (UKIETR), 79, 188
United Nations, 57, 88, 90, 98
United States Air Force, 52, 62
University College Hospital, London, 39
University Hospital, Sarajevo, 57, 91
University of California, Los Angeles, 138
University of Harvard, USA, 143
University of Surrey, 151
University of Zambia, 151
University of Zigazag, Egypt, 141

Vasa, Drs Sanjiv and Purnima, 136
Villeneuve, Jacques, F1 champion, 111
Voodoo, 77

Walker, Murray, OBE, F1 commentator, 111
Wallace, A.B., 19
Wallace, Andy, Le Mans winner, 110

Walsh, Tim, 83
War Crimes Tribunal, The Hague, 99
Waring, Prof. Michael, 174
Watts, Andy, 41
Wessex, The Countess of, 119
West, Sgt Maj., 45
Wexham Park Hospital, 18
Wheatcroft, Tom, 113
White, Maj. Gen. Sir Martin and Lady
 Fiona, 119, 126, 182
Whiteley, Roger, 50
Wilcox, Desmond, 159
Wild Frontiers, 101
Wimbledon Hospital, Haiti, 75
Wimbledon Lawn Tennis
 Championships, 120
Windsor Castle, 56, 124
Wood, Dr Fiona, Australia, 132
Wood, Dr Ian, 21, 175
Worcester College, Oxford, x
Wright, Dr Gordon, Cambridge, 151
Wrightington Hospital, 26
Wrigley, Dr Fenella, 121

Yorkshire, 14
Young, Carol, SJA, 126

Zatriqui, Drs Violeta and Sender, 102